BANFEBA

BANFEBA MEDITATION

SEVEN
ESSENTIAL
STEPS TO
ENLIGHTENMENT

BRUCE
MACWILLIAMS

Copyright © 2018 Bruce MacWilliams

The moral right of the author has been asserted.

Apart from any fair dealing for the purposes of research or private study, or criticism or review, as permitted under the Copyright, Designs and Patents Act 1988, this publication may only be reproduced, stored or transmitted, in any form or by any means, with the prior permission in writing of the publishers, or in the case of reprographic reproduction in accordance with the terms of licences issued by the Copyright Licensing Agency. Enquiries concerning reproduction outside those terms should be sent to the publishers.

Matador
9 Priory Business Park,
Wistow Road, Kibworth Beauchamp,
Leicestershire. LE8 0RX
Tel: 0116 279 2299
Email: books@troubador.co.uk
Web: www.troubador.co.uk/matador
Twitter: @matadorbooks

ISBN 978 1789015 478

British Library Cataloguing in Publication Data.
A catalogue record for this book is available from the British Library.

Printed and bound in Great Britain by 4edge Limited
Typeset in 11pt Minion Pro by Troubador Publishing Ltd, Leicester, UK

Matador is an imprint of Troubador Publishing Ltd

For my son, Weston;
wife, Sheila
& dog, Riley

Contents

INTRODUCTION
The Genesis of This Book　　　　　　ix

Chapter One
ENLIGHTENMENT
BANFEBA MEDITATION　　　　　　1

Step One
BREATHE　　　　　　12

Chapter Two / Step Two
ACCEPT　　　　　　22

Chapter Three / Step Three
NOW　　　　　　38

Chapter Four / Step Four
FEEL　　　　　　59

Chapter Five / Step Five
EXPERIENCE　　　　　　80

Chapter Six / Step Six
BEING   99

Chapter Seven / Step Seven
AWARENESS   107

Chapter Eight
THE SEVEN STEPS   112

Chapter Nine / Seven Results
PERFECT HEALTH
BEAUTY
PROSPERITY
FULFILLMENT
PEACE
LOVE
BLISS   136

EPILOGUE   170

NOTES   175

INTRODUCTION

THE GENESIS OF THIS BOOK

My name is Bruce MacWilliams. My professional career is being a filmmaker, but my paramount goal in life has always been to become enlightened.

I've always wanted to become totally awake to higher states of consciousness. I have been practicing meditation extensively for more than forty years.

I have also studied the lives and works of many great spiritual teachers. They have inspired me, but I have never felt the need to try to join their ranks. In fact, it has never been my outward intention to be a spiritual teacher, but recently everywhere I am I find myself in a deep conversation with old friends, and new friends, who are all headed in a similar spiritual direction, and I seem to have acquired a distinctive voice they are eager to listen to.

On my path to enlightenment, I have discovered a unique meditation technique, *BANFEBA Meditation*. This unique meditation technique has worked very well for me to obtain a higher level of consciousness I describe as a profound awareness of the absolute source of all creation: Being. As a result of my awareness of Being, and my connection to it, the life I have desired to live, filled with good health, beauty, prosperity, fulfillment, peace, love, and bliss – I am now living. I feel this meditation technique is a special gift I was given. I have written this book to share this unique meditation technique, BANFEBA, with the world.

The Beginning

It was the spring of 1974. I was fifteen years old. I was attending the first of four years at Phillips Academy, a prep school, in Andover, Mass. The sun was setting, and I was walking into the Commons building for dinner. Dinner was always a big deal in prep school, despite the horrendous food, because the social magnetism pulled us all in from across the vast campus like determined ants marching to an abandoned cube of sugar. Our sugar was the desire to laugh, joke, share our stories, and of course flirt in that awkward teenage way, where one look or a smile could last in our memory for days; a kiss, or any possible hint of sex, could be reminisced for a lifetime.

Phillips Academy, "Andover", was not your typical high school. It was the Harvard of high schools filled with intelligent, creative, preppie kids on the fast track to higher achievement. It was, and continues to be, an excellent school. We were all very fortunate to attend Andover. Many of our parents were affluent and successful, and we were all raised to continue on that path. My roommate, Will, was President Truman's grandson. Across the hall, my friend Tommy's father was the Prime Minister of Bermuda. By senior year, my first Andover girlfriend, Jenny, had a new boyfriend named John F. Kennedy Jr., and the history of Andover alumni, going all the way back to George Washington's nephew, attested to the fact that an Andover education provided a major opportunity. We were taught achievement and success were paramount objectives in life. If we were willing and able to stay on track, work hard, and go on to an Ivy League University or a top school like Stanford, success was almost guaranteed to be our reward. Fortunately, the founders of Andover were enlightened enough to see beyond only the primary objective of success and achievement. Andover is not just a bunch of rich, spoiled kids. The founding mission of the school is: "Non Sibi" (Not for Oneself) and "Youth From Every Quarter." Andover works very hard to give back to the world through many altruistic school programs and to completely diversify the student body. A large percentage of the students are on scholarship. Andover is the fast track for many, and so much more than just a ticket to an Ivy League University.

Of course, it was 1974 in America, and some of us were teetering on that fast track. We didn't really understand we were on it. We were experimenting with anything exciting and new we could get our hands on, rebelling against the status quo. We wobbled as we went, always about to fall. Andover is a liberal boarding school, and although the academic demands were strict, the social demands were not. We wore long hair, torn jeans, t-shirts, and sneakers to class. A lot of our teachers either didn't know it, or looked the other way, but we were all experimenting with drugs and alcohol. We had grown up watching the Vietnam War on the nightly news, and our politics were mostly liberal. Loud rock music and the smell of burning cannabis were an integral part of our newly created preppie-hippie landscape.

I had worked hard to get into Andover. The admissions process was, and continues to be, extremely competitive, but after I was accepted, I was on cruise control and explore mode. Two close friends were on the same rebellious teenage trajectory, and they didn't make it past the first term. Both were expelled for "experimenting" a little too much. I had been experimenting too, and I was brought in for questioning. They either couldn't prove I had broken the rules, or they were giving me an extra chance because my older brother, John, had excelled at Andover, and he was on his way to Stanford, but the writing was on the wall – it was only my first year, and already my days at Andover were numbered.

On that evening as I entered Commons, I stopped in the doorway, glued to his bright eyes. There was a poster of Maharishi Mahesh Yogi, an Indian guru. I was curious. I had never focused on a picture of a guru before. I grew up a casual Episcopalian, only going to church on holidays and an occasional Sunday. Religion was not part of my life, and I had spent very little time in any kind of spiritual contemplation. Plus, my parents were fairly conservative, and anything that even hinted of a cult was considered completely taboo. Still, I was glued to his eyes. They had a sparkle to them that was unique and hard to explain.

The river of a thousand students rushing to enter the building for dinner was tough to fight, but I stood my ground in the doorway, and I read the poster. It was introducing a lecture on Transcendental Meditation. I asked a few fellow students, as they squeezed past if they knew anything about this event. The first reply was Maharishi was the guru who taught the Beatles to meditate. I always liked the Beatles, so I took the remark as a positive endorsement. Then an older student, a skeptic, walked past and warned me that Maharishi was probably some con man or a cult leader, and to beware. I had always been an adventurous kid, so the hint of danger probably encouraged me to explore further as much as the association with the Beatles.

Two nights later, I navigated my way to the introductory lecture. I sat in the back row. I was skeptical of this "scientifically validated" meditation technique that promised to awaken one to higher states of consciousness, but my intuition told me to at least check it out. There were about a hundred and fifty people in the introductory lecture. Maharishi was nowhere in sight. Instead, a nerdy looking guy, who had the demeanor of a chemistry student from MIT, ranted for about an hour and a half about the effectiveness of Transcendental Meditation (TM). He enumerated all of the numerous scientific studies, conducted at top universities, proving without a doubt TM was extremely good for your health. The next night in the follow-up, preparatory lecture, the same guy went into even more detail. There were about thirty interested students left, and of those thirty only about seven of us took the bait and signed up to learn this "scientifically proven," meditation technique. My continuing curiosity, plus a subtle inherent desire to truly discover something profound, kept leading me forward.

It was a rainy afternoon, and I had to trek all the way across campus bringing with me thirty dollars, a handkerchief, a piece of fruit, and some flowers. I felt a little uncool to be bringing these obscure items to the initial lesson, but the TM teacher, the same guy who gave both lectures, told me it was all part of an ancient Vedic ritual called a Puja, and it had been done this way for thousands of years.

When he lit some incense and started chanting in Sanskrit while bowing to a framed photo of Maharishi, and his teacher, Guru Dev, and the lineage of teachers before them, alarms immediately went off in my head, and I completely felt I had been conned out of my thirty dollars. But I was the only one in the room with the teacher, so there was no one to ridicule me. I had already forked over the cash so I decided just to let go, and see what would happen next.

He gave me a mantra. A mantra is a Sanskrit word that has no meaning to you unless you understand Sanskrit, which few in the West do. We were taught by the TM teacher the mantra was just a sound with a certain vibrational frequency. When the mantra was thought silently, it would allow one to transcend thinking to become aware of higher states of consciousness.

I sat down in a big leather chair in an empty room that looked like it was the old study of a retired professor or an abandoned private library. The TM teacher left me alone and told me to meditate for about twenty minutes. I started to effortlessly think the mantra as instructed. After about four or five minutes, I stopped thinking completely. I dropped into an extremely deep state of awareness. I was completely relaxed, and totally at peace. Never before in my life had I experienced anything even close to that. The peaceful space surrounding me was so thick I could literally feel it. I felt totally encapsulated by a deep, profound silence, and the warm glow of pure love. Instantly, I knew without a doubt; I was in the absolute presence of God.

The rain had stopped. I walked back to my dorm. I felt so incredibly high. I was so clear-headed and awake. It was as if someone had cleaned off my dirty eyeballs, and I was now seeing crystal clear for the first time. The colors were so vibrant and saturated. I could see every detail of the raindrops on the leaves. And all I could think was if meditation was this fantastic, why had I been wasting so much of my time smoking marijuana? This experience was what I had been looking for.

That day I committed to meditating twenty minutes, twice a day, each day for the next four years. By the time I graduated from Andover, I was on three varsity sports, I was elected one of the five student presidents of the school, and I had fallen in love with photography. I gave all the credit to meditation, and I was convinced without it, none of these achievements would have been possible. In fact, I probably wouldn't have made it through the first year. Of course, using meditation as a technique to successfully achieve is a limited perspective. It feels good to succeed, but the fulfillment of success is only temporary. Like most people on Earth, I have spent most of my life continually learning this profound lesson. Later on my journey, I would discover so much more.

By my sophomore year at Cornell University, I was still meditating each day, but the effects had dulled considerably. I

Introduction

had abandoned smoking marijuana, but I was still periodically drinking alcohol. I was young, and it was hard not to enjoy partying in my free time like the rest of the students.

It was springtime again. I was on the Cornell Varsity B Lacrosse team, and we had just finished our last game of the season. I had also just finished my last final exam. I was free for the summer, and I was happy to celebrate with my friends, so I did. The first few beers didn't even faze me. I had been playing and training for the last two years on one of the top lacrosse teams in the country, and I was physically in the best shape of my life. I downed the beers fast and barely felt them.

Then we started drinking tequila, and I should've known better because the only other time I had drunk tequila was the time I was visiting one of my best friends, David Wilson, at the University of Southern California in Los Angeles, and we drank a whole bottle of tequila before a Grateful Dead concert. We had great seats in the seventh row, but we both completely passed out during one of Jerry Garcia's notoriously long guitar solos. I should have learned then. Tequila is beyond alcohol. It is a super-alcohol. But that spring night at Cornell was special. It was the end of the school year. We felt we deserved to live life to the fullest, and we drank accordingly to celebrate.

It was after midnight. We were leaving a bar downtown, following my roommate's friend to a party back on campus. I was driving fast downhill with my good friend and roommate, David Buck. There was a friend of David's in the back seat. It was the first time I had met her. David and I had gone to Andover together. We knew each other well. He cheered me on as our speed increased. His enthusiasm was infectious. David loved to party. He was fearless, and in that exact moment I also felt invincible. I saw his friend, driving in front of us, slow his car down, and put on his turn signal. I thought he was signaling to park on the right side of the road, and I accelerated to pass him on the left, but at the last second he turned left instead. I must've been going about sixty when my car hit the front of his car. My car flipped twice, end over end, and crashed head first, upside down, into a telephone pole. Lights went out; I was unconscious. The car was crumpled like an aluminum can stomped on by a heavy boot. Blood was everywhere.

If you had met me at that stage in my life, previous to the accident, you might have liked me if you had the insight to see past my rebellious arrogance that was trying desperately to cover my youthful insecurities, but for most people my competitive outward nature most likely prevailed, and I am not sure I was particularly amiable. In many ways, I needed a swift kick in the pants, but that night I got a lot more than that.

The police called my parents. My parents called the hospital, and the doctor told my dad it was a fifty-fifty chance I would survive. They immediately hopped on a plane in Philadelphia, and they flew up to the hospital in Syracuse, New York.

David was in even worse shape. He had slipped into a coma, and they weren't sure he would recover. Thank God David's friend in the backseat was fine, and she walked away from the accident. Everyone in the other car was also fine and, thankfully, they walked away from the accident too.

It was 1979, and very few people were driving wearing seatbelts back then. Luckily, that night I was, or I certainly would be dead. The engine came up right into my seat, broke my leg, tore my Achilles tendon, smashed my nose, and ruptured several internal organs. When I came out of the operating room after eight hours of surgery, I was still unconscious, and I was still in critical condition. When I finally awoke, I was in tremendous pain. I have never had thoughts of suicide. I have always been a happy person, but for one second while fighting excruciating pain, I had the thought, "Oh, God, I don't even want to be here."

In that second, I left my body, and I traveled up into a tunnel of white light. It was extremely bright. There were beautiful little angels leading the way. The feeling was so amazing, blissful, and deeply peaceful. It is a secret to most people, but death feels so good you don't want to come back. However, I looked at the bright opening at the other end of the tunnel, which I was floating toward, and I had the thought, "No, I can't go yet. I want to go back. There are things I want to do. I want to help the world." And with that thought, I slipped back into my broken body. I forced my eyes open to see my parents, and my older brother, John, standing over me staring, with looks of pity, at my smashed body and face. Ironically, my near-death experience had left me feeling higher than a kite. At that exact moment, the accident felt like a gift.

I recovered remarkably fast due to my initially strong physical condition, but they hadn't told me how severe David's condition was. They wanted to protect me emotionally and allow me to heal, but as I was getting ready to leave the hospital, they rolled me in a wheelchair to David's room, where he still lay in a coma. When I saw him and realized he might never come back, I cried profusely, and a tremendous feeling of remorse and guilt overwhelmed me. I knew I was responsible. We had all been drinking, but I had been driving.

I spent the summer recuperating physically, but emotionally, I was a total mess. I retreated from my family and friends. I felt like an alien, completely separate from everyone else. I could talk to no one. I meditated as much as possible, and I prayed constantly. I pleaded with God to please let David live. Please bring him back. I promised I would do anything. Take me instead; I'll trade places, or I will spend the rest of my life in your service if only you would let him live.

At the end of the summer, God answered my prayers, and David came out of his coma. He had a few physical complications that took a long time to heal, but overall he was the same guy. He recovered. He left the hospital, and he eventually moved out West to live with his brother in Seattle. I eventually moved down to New York City, so we didn't see each other much after the accident. Life had taken us in different directions, but I remained fond of David. We occasionally talked on the phone, and I always wished him the very best.

David ended up dying several years later. I was told it was due to liver complications from severe drinking, and it was not directly related to the accident. In retrospect, I now realize David had been an alcoholic ever since Andover, even before the accident. At Cornell, I used to watch him drink straight from a bottle of vodka or gin like it was water, and although I thought it was excessive; we all grew up in a culture inundated with drugs and alcohol, so at the time I didn't think too much about it. I did warn him several times to slow down on the drinking, but at that stage in my life, I knew nothing of how addiction worked.

Most of our parents were unaware of our drug and drinking abuse because they were so busy getting drunk themselves. They did it very stylishly, of course, drinking martinis, while dressed formally wearing ties, jackets, and designer dresses, but the truth is – daily, they got smashed. I love both of my parents very much. They were loving, benevolent parents, but the pervasiveness of alcohol was the Achilles heel of the culture they grew up in. Everybody drove drunk in those days. By today's DWI standards they were drunk returning to work after drinking at lunch. They were drunk after "cocktail hour" before dinner, and if there was a party, or a dinner out at a restaurant, they drove home drunk.

I returned to Cornell in the fall after the accident. I was still limping, and I couldn't play lacrosse. I had suffered from a severe concussion, and at first, I could barely concentrate on my studies. I was nervous, thinking it would continue, but through meditation and persistence, I slowly healed.

After my junior year I left Cornell, moved for two years to Newport, Rhode Island, and I worked as a carpenter, builder, and an architect. Then I moved to New York City. I completed my undergraduate Cornell BA degree at Columbia University where I started studying filmmaking. My near-death experience had put me on the fast track spiritually, and I continued to meditate every day as I had since I was 15, but now I was looking for a way to expedite my awakening. It's hard to explain, but when I saw angels first hand, and I believed I had actually spoken to God, I wanted more because I was certain there is much more to life.

I left New York for the weekend, taking the train up to New Haven, Connecticut adjacent to Yale University. I was headed to my first meditation retreat where there were extended periods of meditation lasting several hours. The teachers of the course were surprised this was only my first meditation retreat considering I had already been meditating daily for ten years. I didn't want to insult them, but the real reason was that I was still slightly paranoid about possibly being controlled by a cult. Transcendental Meditation is not a cult. In fact, I highly recommend their meditation technique, but I was still only 25, and I had no outside guidance I trusted, and my family was always very skeptical. Although, eventually each of them, including my parents, gave it a try.

It was at the end of my second meditation session, the afternoon of the second day. I had an extremely unique spiritual experience. I had been meditating several hours that morning, and all day the day before. I came out of meditation, and I immediately fell asleep. I am not sure how long I slept, but suddenly I was completely awake within my body, but my body was still totally asleep. It was as if I were a remote control camera inside my body. I could see my internal organs, my stomach, and my lungs. Then I had the brief thought, "I wonder if I can leave my body?" The next second, that is exactly what I did; I left my body. I went up to the ceiling in the corner of the room, and I looked down on my body sleeping in the bed below. Then I wondered, "Can I go through the wall and leave the house?" And that is exactly what I did. I went through the wall, and I soared up into the afternoon sky. I flew up into the clouds, and way beyond. Then I thought, "I better get back before some other soul takes my body."

I had heard that theory someplace, somewhere before. My concern sent me back down to the house, into the room, and back into my body. When I returned, I was still awake in my sleeping body. Then I thought, "I wonder if I can wake up?" And that is what I did.

That evening before dinner, the teachers of the course asked for our observations on our meditation sessions. I told the teachers, and the assembled course participants, about my incredible experience, and their jaws all dropped. Very few meditators I have known have had such extraordinary experiences. That has never been the goal of meditation, but it was rather surprising, and everyone was definitely intrigued.

The next day before I left, a Ph.D. neuroscientist and research fellow from Harvard Medical School, who was very big in the TM organization showed up, and he asked me a lot of questions about my unique meditation experience. He checked my blood pressure, eyesight, and a few other simple tests. He was a nice guy. His name was Tony Nader. After Maharishi Mahesh Yogi died in 2008, Tony would be named the head of the worldwide TM Movement. He is now called Maharaja Adhiraj Rajaraam.

Back in New York City, my spiritual experiences returned to become fairly normal, and as a film director, I was busy trying to launch my first movie. I wanted to learn the advanced techniques of Transcendental Meditation called the TM-Sidhi program, but it was expensive, and I didn't have the money.

I signed up anyway, and sure enough, the Universe sent it to me. I raised enough money to direct my first movie through courageous investors on Wall Street, and my fee for writing and directing allowed me to take the advanced meditation course.

My experience of the TM-Sidhi technique was astonishing, but it was also slightly bizarre. The last part of the technique, which uses Patanjali's ancient Vedic Sutras, includes a flying sutra at the end of the program. When I practiced the program, I literally lifted off the ground like a frog leaping into the air. I was sitting in a lotus yoga position, and I hopped into the air. It was an awkward jump, but I experienced waves of bliss shooting through my body, and it felt completely effortless.

After I learned the TM-Sidhi technique, I continued to execute it with ease for many years, but I was always just hopping. I was not actually flying or levitating. However, I remember, vividly, on one occasion sitting in lotus yoga position in a sea of over a thousand meditators during a massive meditation assembly. We were in an immense convention room at the Washington Hilton Hotel in Washington DC (where President Reagan was shot a few years earlier in 1981). I was sitting next to a guy from the Caribbean, who I watched with my own two eyes, lift off the ground about three feet in the air, and hang there for at least three seconds before dropping back to the floor. He defied gravity, as we usually know it, and I was utterly amazed. But even that unique experience was not as remarkable as what happened next on my spiritual journey.

It was several years later in 1989. I had reached a crossroads in my life, and I needed direction. I was thirty years old, and I had finished writing and directing my first movie, *Real Cowboy*. We shot it in the South Bronx of New York and Douglas, Arizona. It turned out pretty well. It got distributed, and I was invited to the Cannes Film Festival to showcase it there. It was an exhilarating time. I flew in a chartered jet to France with many other New

York filmmakers, and I was able to meet one of my heroes, Jim Jarmusch, who had directed a movie a few years before, that had inspired me to be a film director, called *Stranger than Paradise*.

When I got to Cannes it was very exciting. I was meeting big directors and attending screenings and parties. Steven Soderbergh was there with his movie, *Sex, Lies and Video Tape*. Spike Lee was there with *Do the Right Thing*. My film didn't get the same enormous reception theirs did, but I had shot it in three weeks on a total budget of $200,000, and I was just happy to be screening my movie in Cannes.

However, when I got back to New York, the party ended. I realized although my movie was sold in territories in the Far East, and parts of Europe, no one in America really saw it, except friends in private screenings. I was back struggling to get my next movie going.

I was also still avidly searching, trying to find a clearer, higher high through meditation. I went on another meditation retreat. In these retreats, especially now that I was practicing the TM-Sidhi technique, I was doing extended programs that were more advanced. The puja ceremonies I witnessed were getting stranger with a lot more religious connotations. By that point, even though the TM organization still claimed Transcendental Meditation was a scientifically proven technique, with no overt religious association, I had discovered the mantras we were using in our meditation practice were the Sanskrit names of Hindu deities.

Now, the Transcendental Meditation technique was still working, and it has been scientifically proven advantageous in numerous studies, but for one moment one night, when I got back to New York City on the train, after another weekend in Connecticut of meditating extensively, I was in the process of releasing a lot of built-up stress, and I felt very skeptical, and cynical. I wasn't adverse to the Hindu religion or any other religion. I have close friends with all different religious backgrounds, but I was baptized an Episcopalian, and for some reason that night I felt paranoid. I was also paranoid about my future as a filmmaker. Intuitively, I knew I was at a crossroads, and I went to sleep that night asking God for guidance.

I awoke in my bed in the middle of the night. I opened my eyes and looked to the doorway of my bedroom. The room was dark, but standing in the entrance was a man. I received him without any fear. Instead, a very warm feeling of love surrounded me. The man glowed, emanating an intense white light. I looked closer, and I instantly realized, with absolutely no doubt – he was Jesus Christ.

The words he spoke to me were sent telepathically. I could hear him clearly, but his lips never moved. He said to me, "You are on the right path. Stay on it. Do not be afraid. I will watch over you. I am always with you."

I instantly understood my direction in life. All of my questions were answered. I just watched him for as long as I could. The love, happiness, and peace I felt were beyond words. Slowly, I slipped back into a deep sleep with Jesus still standing there, watching over me.

I awoke the next morning, and I bolted straight up in bed. Was that real? Did that really happen? Was I dreaming? No, I was not dreaming. It was perfectly clear. I was completely awake. It really did happen. I have told very few people in my life that story. It is the most special moment of my life, tied for first place with the birth of my son, Weston.

Is it hard to believe? Yes, but as you discover your own profound connection to the absolute source of all creation, God, I call Being, I have a strong, visceral sense you will believe more. A powerful positive energy is filling my body as I write these words, confirming we are both on the right path. Let's begin.

Chapter One

ENLIGHTENMENT

Enlightenment is the awakening of our awareness to the point at which we recognize and allow the continual experience of a higher level of consciousness. That experience of a higher level of consciousness can be described as a total union with the Source of all creation, God, or Being. Ultimately, however, our experience will be personal, and we can use any description that suits us.

An enlightened state of higher consciousness is experienced as freedom from fears and doubts, a feeling of deep peace, intense happiness, unlimited love, complete fulfillment, and a profound connection with everyone and everything that exists in the Universe. This higher level of consciousness is beyond a complete explanation; only our personal experience can entirely describe it to us, but as we start experiencing it more and more we will begin to understand, emphatically, the journey of life is truly all about becoming awake to what we really are – a divine soul with infinite potential.

BANFEBA MEDITATION

BANFEBA Meditation is a unique meditation technique comprised of Seven Essential Steps, that will allow you to experience the sequential awakening of enlightenment. BANFEBA Meditation is a powerful and dynamic form of meditation because it can be practiced throughout the day, every day, and that extended experience of Being will dramatically expedite the process of enlightenment.

BANFEBA also works very well in conjunction with Vedic Mantra Meditation, and Yogic breathing techniques. Your present religion or belief system will only be further supported by BANFEBA, and in no way does this meditation technique interfere with your current practice. BANFEBA will help you, regardless of your own direction in life, to become more awake, and evolved.

My personal spiritual journey has been the catalyst of my discovering the BANFEBA Meditation technique. I had been meditating extensively for forty years using Vedic mantra meditation (TM), and the results were beneficial, but I wanted more. Deep in meditation, I asked God for guidance. BANFEBA Meditation was the answer. The Seven Steps: Breathe, Accept, Now, Feel, Experience, Being, Awareness allowed me to become totally awake to the inherent source of who we all are – Being.

Being

Most people still envision their lives are confined to what happens to them individually – separate from others, separate from the whole. Most people, therefore, only experience a tiny fraction of what they really are. We are not just these little people walking around in these little separate bodies. We are connected and part of everything in the Universe because our core is the same as the core of the Universe. That core is Being.

The Goal of Life is to Reach Enlightenment

As an individual person here on Earth, we may think the goal of life is to live to the fullest, stay healthy, have a rewarding career, become wealthy, fall in love, and raise a happy family. Yes, those are all worthy goals, and we can continue to achieve them or other specific personal goals we have chosen, but ultimately, the number one goal is the same for all of us whether we recognize it or not. That goal is to become enlightened – to become awake to and continually experience Being.

Innately, we know this is true on a visceral level because nothing else, alone, will completely satisfy us. Nothing, no matter how great it may seem theoretically, will ultimately, continually, satisfy us when we achieve or receive it. *The fulfillment of success is temporary.* We will always want more, constantly delaying our happiness, never feeling fulfilled – until we are enlightened.

Ironically, if we make the goal of reaching enlightenment, our primary goal all of our other goals will be significantly easier to achieve. The more awake we become to our direct connection to the Source of all creation, the more all situations in life we desire will be created. We will be able to achieve our goals. We must always remember, however, that the fulfillment we gain from achieving those goals is only temporary.

The infinite correlation of all things and events within the Universe is extremely complex and, honestly, beyond the human mind to totally comprehend. It is impossible to totally understand infinite possibilities. There are theories in quantum physics pointing us in the right direction, and we can understand specific laws of nature, etc., but valid or not, theories alone will most likely only lead to more debate.

The only way to completely understand and believe what is expressed about the subject of enlightenment is to have the actual experience.

One quick experience of pure consciousness will be enough to attract similar awakened experiences. Expansion of our awareness will continue until a full awakening occurs. The direct, tangible experience of Being is totally, completely enlightening because Being is the absolute source of everything in the Universe.

Enlightenment and God

The word, God, has so many connotations and a variety of meanings to different people. Some teachers believe those associations slow down a true understanding and experience of enlightenment, and they chose to use other descriptions. Your experience of the Source, the state of pure consciousness, a feeling of deep peace, and unlimited love, is unique for you. Call that experience anything you want. You may not prefer the word, God; you might call it, the Absolute, the Source, the Now. It is your prerogative to chose the description that feels right for you.

Some people may associate the experience with a religious expression: Christ Light, Jesus, Abraham, Buddha, Krishna, Rama, Muhammad, Allah, or many other names. Those words and other names connected to the Source all work for me, too. The actual feeling and experience will be similar, regardless of what we call it.

It is time to get past words, or any perceived religious or spiritual differences. Any of the great, master spiritual teachers throughout history would advise we unite now at this crucial stage of our evolution. Enlightenment is the goal for us all irrespective of the words we use to describe it. When we experience the tangible feeling of Being on a regular basis, we will naturally be led directly to enlightenment regardless of what we call it.

Spiritual Terminology

As we study both ancient spiritual and modern New Age teachers on our road to enlightenment, we will read and hear different terminology basically explaining the same experience. It can be confusing if we are looking for an exact language to express what really is a subjective feeling.

Throughout history, people have fallen victim to the confusion of certain dogmas, jargon, and belief systems whether it is from an ancient religion or a modern spiritual movement. It is time we each come to the simple and yet profound truth – we don't need to follow a certain doctrine, dress, or act a certain way, or follow any special rituals to become enlightened.

Jesus was teaching us to become enlightened two thousand years ago, but the language he used confuses many today, because words, and their meaning change over time with many translations compounding the problem. We must respect all ancient religions and belief systems for maintaining enough knowledge to keep the quest of enlightenment alive, but as a species, we also need to continue to evolve. We need to stay awake to what those great teachers were trying to allow us to actually experience.

Once again, our actual experience is really the only true teacher. Words will only point us in the direction of that experience. The goal is to have the actual experience of enlightenment.

Being is Absolute

As we become more awake, more aware, more enlightened, our actual experience of Being becomes clearer. Our world then literally changes because our individual worlds are merely reflections of our individual states of consciousness. Being, however, is absolute and doesn't change or expand. Being already encompasses infinite possibilities; there is no need to expand.

Through our personal awakening, our expansion of awareness, we are able to see that our connection with the Source has always been there. We already are expressions of God. *It is only our perception that changes.* We only need to become awake to that reality for us to start experiencing it. Once that happens, significant changes in our lives will occur.

Being is Your Soul

Your soul is your individual awareness of Being. Your soul is your Higher Self. Enlightenment is your Higher Self, your soul, becoming awake to itself, Being.

Reality of Unity

Once our awareness starts to become more awake on the path to enlightenment, our experience will expand accordingly, our lives will change in a dynamically positive way, and we will begin to see the interconnectedness of everything. It is awe-inspiring how fast a person's life can change once they start to experience higher states of consciousness, once they become cognizant of their innate connectedness with everything in the infinite Universe.

Enlightenment is a real, tangible experience. Enlightenment is the awakening of our physical awareness to be able to feel, see, taste, hear, and understand we are not only this sole individual walking around Earth in this singular body; we are entirely connected and part of everything in the infinite Universe.

Enlightened Creation

Because we already are connected with the Source of all creation, we actually are now creating the world we live in. It is an inherent process we may not be aware of, but it is, nevertheless, still happening. Everything in the Universe reflects our unique perception of it. *The combined perception of the collective consciousness of humanity creates the world we live in today.*

Good, Bad, Right and Wrong

The Source, God, is not Santa Claus. God has absolutely no judgment in whether we have been good, bad, right or wrong in our life. If we have been discharging negative thoughts, actions, and energy into the Universe, that energy has linked up to the exact degree with similar energy and expressed itself in our life. If we have gone far enough in a negative direction – our lives can be thought of as living in hell. However, we are only one experience away from completely changing our direction, and turning our lives completely around to the point we can now literally live a life of Heaven on Earth. *Always remember, we are brand new every second, and absolutely perfect, right now.*

Experience is Your Teacher

You need not have faith in these words that you can create Heaven on Earth. Words are only seeds of knowledge. You need the actual experience to fully awaken. This theme will be repeated many times because you must become awake to the process of letting your experience teach you how to reach enlightenment. Experience is your teacher on the path to enlightenment.

Words are only indicators of the direction we should head. We have to pick a direction and head toward enlightenment. Our own experience will teach us if that direction works for us. We are, each of us, ultimately, the primary teachers on our spiritual journeys. This book is merely a road sign, pointing you down a specific path. It is a good path, but it is always your choice which direction you will go, and how fast you will reach enlightenment.

Igloo in the Sun

Imagine for an instant; you have lived your entire life alone on a small deserted island in the Caribbean. You have grown up in a small hut made of wood on the beach. You never have had any access to the outside world – no mail service, no TV, no phone, no cell phone, no computer, Internet, Skype, Facebook, Twitter, or Instagram. You don't even have any books or magazines. You have nothing mechanical or electric on the island – no stove, no fridge, no AC, no car, nothing. You only know the very small, simple world you live in.

Suddenly, a distant cousin you have never met before, and you didn't even know existed, lands on your island in his private jet. It was a tricky landing on a dirt road in the middle of a sugar cane field, but your cousin's pilot is exceptional, and he landed effortlessly.

That night, sitting at a fire on the beach in front of your hut, eating dinner, you ask your cousin to tell you where he is from. He tells you he is an Eskimo, and he has lived his whole life in an igloo at the North Pole. Until recently when British Petroleum discovered oil on his patch of ice, and he instantly became exceedingly wealthy. He bought a Gulfstream private jet, and he is now flying around the world to discover the truth of life. (We're hoping he also learns how to leave a smaller environmental footprint, but that is another story.)

It all sounds totally ludicrous to you. You didn't even know there was a world out there to explore. You have never seen anything beyond your island. So you start asking him questions, and your first question is – what is an igloo? Your cousin explains it is a house made of snow. So you ask him, what is snow? He looks out at the ocean pounding on the beach in front of you both, and he says snow is water that becomes very cold. You look at him like he is completely nuts. You ask him again – are you saying you live in a house made of water? And he responds: yes, very cold water. He tries to explain it further, but you just can't understand or believe him. It has never dropped below 60 degrees on your island, and you have never experienced snow. You don't exactly fight, but you aren't exactly disheartened, when he takes off in his jet to continue his travels. You think your cousin is insane to believe a house can be made of water, but you can't help but be impressed by the jet.

The next year, he mysteriously shows up again. He would've called first, but you still don't have a phone. He lands again on the island in his jet, but this time he brings with him a portable camping cooler, packed with snow. That night at dinner, he takes the snow out and makes it into a miniature igloo like the one he grew up living in at the North Pole. You are amazed when you see this new cold substance called snow, and even more amazed when it melts by the fire and turns into water.

There is no way to truly believe a house can be made of water until you have experienced snow. Life is like that. We didn't completely believe the world was round until someone sailed to the horizon. We didn't believe we could fly in a plane, until someone did, and we actually saw it happen. Experience is the best teacher.

Repetition

BANFEBA Meditation is a Seven Step technique that allows you to have the actual experience of a higher state of consciousness that will eventually lead you to full enlightenment. Repetition of the Seven Steps helps it become a natural habit so; eventually, you won't have to even think of it for it to become your actual experience; it will be automatic. If you want to do anything in life from learning how to walk to learning how to run a marathon, you need to repeat the steps until they are second nature to you.

The knowledge contained in the Seven Steps will lead you to the experience. In this book, I repeat the knowledge continuously for it to become automatic for you. The knowledge will lead directly to the experience. You need the actual experience of a higher state of consciousness to achieve a state of enlightenment, but don't be intimidated; the experience you are looking for is already within you, and a lot easier to become aware of than you may believe.

Who is Enlightened?

There is no definite way to know whether anyone else is enlightened or not, and really no need to know. Our egos love to compare and compete, but we shouldn't fall into that trap, it will only slow down our awakening. We can see the sparkle in someone's eyes reflecting within him or her a vast infinite source of energy, but it could easily fade if they get caught in a cycle of thinking, and they separate from the Source of their creation. Laughter and bliss are good signs. Maharishi always laughed, had a great sense of humor, and a blissful smile, but it is easy to radiate love when surrounded by so many people that love you. What happens when an enlightened person gets caught in a traffic jam? Is he or she laughing then?

Ultimately, we all live in a relative plane of existence that will fluctuate as we experience it, giving us different experiences, some good, some bad. The distinction of someone who is totally awake in a state of enlightenment is that person is always aware of both the relative plane of existence and Being, the Absolute level of existence that is the source of all creation.

An enlightened person may get caught in a traffic jam too, and they may not initially be laughing or feeling bliss. They may even briefly get angry, but they will also simultaneously be aware of a deep peace within, and the deep peace surrounding them. Through that peaceful feeling, they will start to enjoy whatever situation they are presently in – even being in a traffic jam.

We all have this ability to tap into what is naturally already there in all of us: the absolute peace of Being. Some people are more cognizant of that reality, and they experience it more than others, but ultimately, we are all one big field of energy, united at our core by Being, so it doesn't help to try to differentiate in any way, thinking I am enlightened, and you are not, or you are, and I am not.

"I am enlightened" is a statement made by the ego. That process of thinking only brings about separation. Who is the "I" that is enlightened? Enlightenment is experienced as Unity Consciousness. Unity Consciousness is recognizing and experiencing the oneness of us all. It is inevitable we all will experience a taste of enlightenment at some point. We are all just working out the details on how we each get there. This book is part of that process.

Levels of Enlightenment

Some spiritual teachers from the Vedic tradition that is thousands of years old, considered by many the oldest source of knowledge of humanity, talk about distinct levels of awareness or enlightenment. Maharishi described the different levels of enlightenment as Cosmic Consciousness, God Consciousness, Unity Consciousness, and finally, Brahman Consciousness.

Some Vedic teachers are adamant the levels are distinct, corresponding to different levels of awareness. While this may be interesting to contemplate, there is no exact map to reaching enlightenment, and abiding by a theoretical plan may slow us down in a cycle of thoughts. The key to reaching enlightenment at any level is to transcend our desires and transcend thinking.

We need to transcend cycles of thought and become awake to awareness of Being. Keep it simple, practice BANFEBA Meditation – become aware of and experience Being more each day, and your life will become happier and happier. Remember, only our egos care about levels of achievement. We need to transcend our egos to reach enlightenment.

Step One
BREATHE

Banfeba Meditation

BANFEBA Meditation is a technique comprised of seven steps: *Breathe, Accept, Now, Feel, Experience, Being, Awareness.* These Seven Steps should be practiced assiduously, in quick succession, until they become one effortless simultaneous action. Any coordinated action from pitching a baseball to playing the guitar can be broken down into distinct steps. When the steps are done in effortless synchronization, they flow together as one action. The one action of BANFEBA Meditation is accomplished the same way. *Breathe and Accept the Now; Feel and Experience Being Awareness.*

BANFEBA Meditation is a skill that takes practice to master. Once the distinct steps are understood clearly, practiced, and done in effortless coordination, the steps all become one automatic action without any thinking.

The advantage of BANFEBA Meditation is it can be done with your eyes open or closed at any time throughout the day. You can spend 10 to 20 minutes in a BANFEBA Meditation session with your eyes closed, or you can briefly practice it for only ten to twenty seconds with your eyes open whenever you get the chance.

The First Step; Breathe

The first essential step of BANFEBA Meditation is to breathe deeply through your nose and simply be aware of your breathing. *Breathe deeply through your nose several times to get started then just breathe normally. Follow your own natural pace and rhythm as your breathing naturally slows down. Don't think about your breathing; just simply be aware of your breathing.* Simple, effortless, subtle awareness of your breathing as it slows down combined with the six remaining essential steps of BANFEBA Meditation, after training and practice, will allow the direct experience of Being.

Enlightenment is really only the expanding of your awareness until you experience the tangible *feeling of Being, infinite peace,* and realize it is always there at the core of everything you experience in the relative world. Once you experience Being on a regular basis, the experience will attract more similar experiences, and you will become more aware it is always there. This process is completely natural and very simple, yet, without the right guidance, it is almost impossible to discover.

Become Aware of your Breath to Transcend Thinking

The key to enlightenment is to become aware Being is always at the source of everything in creation. In order to become aware of Being you must transcend your desires. You must transcend your thinking. Transcend your thinking by shifting your awareness to your breathing, and then shifting your awareness from your breathing to Being. *Once you are aware of Being, simultaneously there at the source of your breathing, feel it.* It all starts very simply by directing your attention to your breathing. Become aware of your breath at its most subtle, ethereal level.

Your awareness will naturally expand until you are also aware of Being, absolute silence, in the background of everything all the time.

Stay aware of Being as long as you can. Your awareness will be hijacked by thoughts, and you will lose the awareness of Being. Return your awareness to Being by repeating the process. Become aware of your breathing as it becomes more and more subtle. As this happens, your awareness will naturally expand until you are also aware of Being. At times your breathing may even cease completely. This is fine. You will naturally return to breathing. Stay aware of Being.

Always remember not to become attached to your breathing. *Your breath is only the vehicle; the destination is Being. Once you feel Being, maintain that feeling, by keeping your awareness on Being.* When you notice you are caught again in a cycle of thoughts, return your awareness effortlessly to Being.

Bhagavad-Gita and Einstein

The theme of the *Bhagavad-Gita*, one of the most respected spiritual books from the ancient Vedic tradition, is to remain unattached in life. On a practical level it means transcend your desires. Transcend your thinking. Thinking is what attaches you to life. Move beyond thinking, and you won't attach yourself to the relative world you have created for yourself. You want to transcend your attachment to the relative world because the relative world will always include destruction as part of the cycle of life. Destruction is part of the large cycle of our whole life and the micro, daily, cycle of life. Anger, frustration, fear, and all other negative emotions are part of the small cycle of destruction. The bigger cycle of destruction may include sickness, depression, emotional distress, serious accidents, altercations, financial loss, etc. When we witness destruction at any level from the perspective of Being it does not totally consume us. We still may have to live through it, but it won't destroy us. We recognize destruction is inherent in the cycle of growth and evolution. We remain unattached to the emotional feeling of destruction. It will still bother us, and we will try to remedy the situation, but it does not totally consume us emotionally because when we transcend our desires and our thinking, we are able to feel, and experience the peace and love of Being. We are able to still experience the infinite peace of Being as we witness the destruction.

Our analytical brains are naturally programmed to think. Every inventor and scientist throughout history was "thinking" when he or she discovered his or her incredible invention or major scientific breakthrough, but the analytical mind is needed a lot less than you may believe. Einstein believed true genius just came to him effortlessly in periods of absolute clarity. He may have been thinking for weeks before that period of clarity, but when true inspiration came, it was effortless and absent of thought. This observation provoked Einstein to say, "There is no logical way to the discovery of elemental laws. There is only the way of intuition, which is helped by a feeling for the order lying behind the appearance."[1]

Breathing is your Vehicle to Become Aware of Being

Transcend thinking by shifting your awareness to your breathing. *Awareness of your breathing is your vehicle to awareness of Being.* Keep practicing this first step until you are able to become aware of, and experience the absolute peace of Being, the Source of all creation. The profound feeling of absolute peace is the foundation behind everything at its Source. You will become aware you are part of an amazing world where everything is interconnected by Being.

Beyond thinking is Being, a field of absolute energy and deep silence, so comprehensive it is infinite. It is beyond complete understanding, but every answer to every question lives there.

The field of absolute energy, Being, is the basis of infinite intelligence. Genius lives there. We just have to experience that field, and every answer to every question will be discovered. Ironically, transcending thinking is the only way for us to allow infinite intelligence to express itself.

Yes, we need our thinking minds for practical purposes. Your thinking mind will always be a tool you will continue to use even when you are enlightened, but not to the point it takes control of who you are. When you are enlightened, you will become aware of, and experience, you are not only the personality your mind has created. You are part of something much bigger, something so wondrous and profound; you are part of Being, God.

Breathing; a Natural Technique

Conscious breathing is the perfect vehicle to transcend thinking to experience Being because we are already naturally breathing constantly to sustain life. Because we are constantly breathing, BANFEBA will naturally expedite the experience of enlightenment.

Awareness of Breathing is Profoundly Simple

We want to move beyond thinking because our thinking mind limits us from being aware of Being. Jesus said, "Thy kingdom come. Thy will be done on Earth, as it is in Heaven."[2] The thinking mind blocks us from our ability to be aware that Heaven is right here in the midst of us, and since we are not aware of it, we are not experiencing it.

Breathing meditation techniques have been taught alone and in conjunction with other meditation and yoga techniques for centuries. There are many specific breathing techniques such as Pranayama, and Kriya breathing techniques taught by many great Vedic spiritual teachers. However, we don't need to put breathing techniques into a specific pattern, with a certain number of repetitions and procedures in order to transcend thinking, and sometimes those specific procedures defeat the purpose.

The purpose must always be to move beyond thinking to allow the experience of Being, already there in the background, to become the predominant experience. The breathing should liberate us from our desires. It should liberate us from our thinking, not bind us with more desires and more thinking. Counting or analyzing the breathing procedure is thinking. Thinking leads to more thinking, and that is counterproductive.

Take a deep breath through your nose. You only need to remind yourself to actually do it. When you slip back into thinking, breathe again. Be subtly aware of your breath, but don't think about it. *Breathe in slowly, deeply in through the nose, and naturally, exhale. Become aware of your breathing until it naturally slows down. Become awake to your actual awareness until you are simultaneously aware of the deep silence of Being.* That is the first step to the seven steps of BANFEBA Meditation; there is nothing more to it.

The First Experience of Being is Extremely Subtle

Remember, Being, is always there but you have probably been ignoring it for most of your life so the experience will be extremely subtle at first, almost as if it is hiding. Keep trying to find it. Don't give up. Feel it. It is there, and the more you experience Being, the more it will show itself, and the more profound the experience will become.

Breathe deeply through your nose, shift your awareness to your breathing, as often as you like throughout the day. Feel the subtle energy of Being. Feel the air filling your lungs. Exhale naturally. Follow your own rhythm. Become aware of your breathing naturally slowing down. Your breathing will become more subtle. Your breathing will lead you to the experience of

Being. Our physical bodies are all slightly different. You will find your own pace. Your pace of breathing may change at different times. *Just be natural. Be effortless.*

Becoming aware of your breathing allows you to transcend thinking. *Breathing allows you to follow your awareness naturally to Being.* When you feel a deep peace, you are on track. When you are aware of the absolute silence in the background, that is good. Let your experience teach you. Being is absolute, but as your awareness awakens your experience of Being becomes deeper. Don't judge it; just be aware of it. Enjoy it. Start by breathing; this is the first step. We will build on it, and talk a lot more about conscious breathing as we continue. By the seventh step, it should all come together for you. Don't give up. This is a process. BANFEBA Meditation takes a lot of practice to master, but hang in there – the results will be everything you have ever wanted in life.

Breathe Your Way Into the Zone

I am a writer and a film director. I have written and directed two movies for my love of the art, I have directed many TV commercials to pay my bills, and I have directed many Public Service Announcements (PSA), volunteering my time, to help the world. In December 2007, I directed a PSA to expand public awareness of the atrocities being committed in Darfur and Uganda, where genocide was happening. This horrific situation had gone unnoticed by too many in the world, including me, for too long. I knew very little about it until I was invited to direct this campaign of PSAs by my good friend, producer, and long-term meditator, Hunter Payne, who runs a great non-profit organization called Aid Still Required. Hunter called and told me to get ready because we would be filming the LA Lakers to hopefully bring a lot of public awareness to help the people of Darfur.

ENLIGHTENMENT

We quickly assembled a small crew. We procured a good broadcast quality HD camera, a few Kino Flo lights, a teleprompter, and a soundman. We showed up while the Lakers were practicing at the Toyota Sports Center in Los Angeles. At the end of the practice, members of the press barraged the players with the standard questions of scores, strategies, and team gossip. I directed the crew to set up our camera, lights, and the teleprompter at the other end of the court. The Lakers finished answering questions, and then they escaped to their locker room. The press left, and we continued to prepare. Then Hunter and the Lakers press agent started bringing down the Lakers, one by one, to the end of the court where we were set up.

I would give each player a simple direction. I would tell them to look straight into the camera, which I was operating, and read the lines on the screen in front of the lens, generated by the teleprompter. My simple direction to the players was to say the words from their heart with conviction. It sounds easy, but as anyone knows who has tried to stand in front of a camera and deliver lines, it is a lot more difficult than it seems. There is a reason top actors get paid millions of dollars because like becoming a professional athlete; it is very hard to master. If it were easy, everyone would be doing it.

Kobe Bryant stepped up to the camera, and he shot bullets through his eyes straight at the camera. His performance was absolutely perfect. To my knowledge, he's not an actor, but the same principles of shooting from the line well, and delivering a line well, applies. If we want to be as good as Kobe Bryant or Denzel Washington we've got to be in the Zone. We experience the Zone when we are intrinsically aware of Being.

The Zone is where everything slows down. It is where thoughts are not interrupting your intense focus. It is where hitting a 95 mph fastball or returning a 110 mph tennis serve comes effortlessly. It is a state of awareness where you are not interrupted by the crowd or having thoughts of losing, or fantasies of winning. You are not thinking of what you are going to do with the trophy, or the extra money, as you are lining up a twenty-foot putt.

Brilliant actors like Denzel Washington, Ben Kingsley, Cate Blanchett, and Meryl Streep have all figured out how to stop thinking when they slip into their characters. They are in the Zone. They are in the present moment. They are in the Now.

Numerous professional athletes like Kobe have been using breathing techniques to transcend thinking, slip into the Zone, into the Now, for many years. A lot of these athletes have no knowledge gurus, yogis, and meditation teachers have been teaching this technique for centuries. They just know it works. Next time you watch an NBA game and a player walks up to the foul line to throw, watch him bounce the ball several times to get into the rhythm, then watch him take a *deep breath*, exhale, and shoot.

Next time you watch a pro golfer make a difficult putt, watch him or her breathe deeply first. Watch a Major League Baseball pitcher breathe deeply before a tough pitch. Many top athletes use this technique constantly. Why? Because it works – when you breathe deeply you naturally become aware of Being. When you naturally transcend thinking to experience Being you have momentarily jumped into the driver's seat of all of creation. Being is another name for the Zone. Being is another name for God. God is an excellent pitcher. God never misses a putt. If you can stay in the Zone, you will be on the fast track to whatever greatness you wish to achieve. Conscious breathing is the first step. You breathe to transcend your desires, and ironically, you end up achieving what you desired.

Experience the Zone

How do you know if it is working? You will experience it. It will be very subtle to start, and then it will build. Always remember, let your own personal experience be your teacher. Use BANFEBA as a technique while playing sports, music, creating art, writing, acting, speaking in public, or at work, to get into the Zone and perform at your highest ability.

Consciously Breathe to Experience Being

Breathe deeply, and put your awareness on your breathing until you transcend your desires; until you transcend your cycle of thoughts. Accept the thoughts, but allow your awareness to follow your breath. Breathe deeply until you are aware of and feel the subtle energy shift, until you feel the stressful thinking mind letting go of control, until you feel the soothing absolute peace of pure consciousness, of present moment awareness, of Being.

In the beginning, the thinking mind controlled by your ego will fight hard to stay in control. Your mind will even run interference and dismiss everything else as irrelevant or false, including your breathing technique or the Seven Steps. But your conscious breathing is your weapon to fight back and regain control of who you really are, which is much bigger and greater than your ego and your mind. Breathing is the first essential step to experiencing enlightenment. *Breathe and Accept the Now; Feel and Experience Being Awareness.*

Chapter Two

Step Two:
ACCEPT

Inherit the Earth

When Jesus said, "Blessed are the meek: for they shall inherit the earth,"[3] he was referring to those blessed people who have reached such a deep level of acceptance they are completely living in the present moment; the Now. Their meekness is a description of their deep level of acceptance. Through their total acceptance, they are living in absolute presence. They are, therefore, experiencing life with a total connection to God. God encompasses all of creation, including the earth; hence, through the process of total acceptance, the meek will inherit the earth.

Deep acceptance is where you actually accept the feeling you are experiencing right now, regardless of your situation, and regardless of the initial feeling, without judgment. *Through acceptance, we are able to transcend desires and transcend thinking, to feel and experience Being.* Being is always there in the background ready to transform our reality if we can transcend our attachment to thinking.

Totally Accept; Truly Surrender

Acceptance is a form of surrender that will allow you to transcend your deepest desires and your constant thinking to experience Being. You can't just say to yourself, okay I surrender – *you have to physically feel the surrender* – totally accept the feeling you have right now.

If you are angry, accept the feeling of anger. If you are sad, accept the feeling of sadness. If you are anxious, accept the feeling of anxiety. Don't continue to think how angry, sad, or anxious you are, just accept it, and feel it. Conversely, if you are happy or elated continue to feel that, but don't think about how happy you are either, just feel it. Observe your feeling, witness your feeling, become aware of your feeling without thinking about it.

Remember, we need to transcend all desires and all course of thinking in order to experience Being. Be on guard for thoughts of grandeur, and fantasies of greatness. Those are just more ego induced thought patterns trying to trap us in our ego controlled lower self, and ironically, they will eventually end up leading us to thoughts and feelings of doubt, fear, and despair.

No matter what situation you find yourself in always remember to totally accept the feeling you are presently having. You must transcend your desires. Acceptance will allow you to transcend your desires, and your thoughts, in order to experience Being. *The only feeling, ultimately, leading to lasting contentment is the feeling of Being.*

Accept Your Thoughts to Transcend Your Thoughts

Desires and thoughts will naturally arise at all times in life, even when you are enlightened. Your thinking mind will always be there, and it will always generate thoughts. Thinking is not bad;

it is necessary to think to navigate through life. However, in order to experience more profound levels of Being, we need to transcend thinking. *We must accept our thoughts to transcend our thoughts.* It is a paradox that has confused many, including myself, for a long time.

Being, God, is the Source of all creation. Once something has been created we must accept it. *Acceptance is the key to transcendence.* Accept your thoughts, and you will be able to transcend your thoughts. Conversely, if you fight your thoughts, you will attach yourself to them, and you will not be able to experience Being.

Accept Your Desires to Transcend Your Desires

Desire is the catalyst that fuels thinking. We want this. We want that. We constantly desire something new, because we are not totally happy. We are not fulfilled. The experience of Being is totally fulfilling, but our thoughts, driven by our desires, are keeping us from experiencing Being. The irony of life is in order to experience the absolute peace of fulfillment; we need to transcend all desires including the desire for peace. We need to completely accept the Now. Accept your desires to transcend your desires. When we transcend our desires, when we turn off the desire-machine, we are able to transcend all thinking and experience Being.

Accept Your Ego to Transcend Your Ego

Ultimately, our egos are an illusion. We identify with our thoughts and our desires. That identity becomes our ego. Our egos, which are cycles of thoughts, mostly create our individual personalities. Our egos have their own agenda, and in some ways, we benefit from that plan on our course through life. However, we think our personality is who we actually are, but we are not that; we are much bigger. We are Being. We are Being experiencing itself.

If our egos are not balanced with an awareness of Being, our egos will naturally expand until they are checked by some sort of destruction in our lives. As we become more self-centered and narcissistic we increasingly head towards failure, tragedy, or disease. The ego path naturally leads to destruction. The destruction will consequently subdue the ego so we are redirected to an awareness of Being. That is how nature works. Your Higher Self, God, is always redirecting you towards awareness of who you really are. God is always redirecting you toward enlightenment. Aging is part of the natural process of subduing our egos. In the first part of our lives we may become successful and wealthy. Our ego may expand accordingly, and we feel a high level of confidence. Then as we age, our bodies naturally start to decay, and we begin to feel insecure. Also, eventual failures in life, which are part of the natural cycle of life, will start to temper that confidence.

Awareness of Being is the goal in life, and the ego clouds our perception so we are not awake to that reality until the ego has been diminished. Being will always guide us back to an awareness of Being. Destruction is part of that natural cycle. The key to keeping the ego in balance without having to endure destruction in our lives is to accept the ego in order to transcend it. If we fight the ego it will only reinforce and solidify the ego. If we accept the ego, we transcend the ego, and experience Being. When we are fully aware of Being, nothing can totally pull us away from our experience of Being. *Your Higher Self, Being, will become the source of your awareness.* That is the experience of enlightenment, and your world will reflect that with peace, happiness, and love.

Surfing for Acceptance

Before I was busy being a father and married, I used to surf a lot in my free time with several friends I grew up with. We would wake up very early, and head up the coast of California from Santa Monica where I live to Malibu. We would catch a few waves before the usual crowd of surfers arrived later in the day.

I was an adequate surfer, but surfing was frustrating for me because I never gained the expert level of achievement I did in my favorite sport, skiing. I grew up skiing. I skied a lot, and eventually, I excelled at it. Surfing fulfillment, however, continued to elude me. I grew up surfing on eastern Long Island on the East coast, during the summers, and the waves were inconsistent, so it was hard to practice enough to get good. And when the waves did finally show up, we had to fight for them. My friends and I grew up playing all sports competitively, and surfing was no different. As I grew older, the competitive part of surfing, fighting for the waves, irritated me. I realized the natural, fun part of surfing was being overshadowed by my ego trying to prove I was a great athlete.

Early one foggy morning, two of my life-long friends, the Wilson brothers, and I drove up to Malibu at sunrise to catch a swell that was supposed to be arriving that day. It was a quiet drive up the coast because we hadn't quite woken up yet. We hiked down the canyon, carrying our boards, on the steep dirt path to the beach below. The beach was empty, and the water was calm. There was a fog belt about a quarter mile offshore. The early morning sun was diffused by the fog, and it was fairly dark.

We paddled out into the fog. There seemed to be no waves, and we waited, sitting on our boards in the tranquil water, about thirty feet apart, in silence. Suddenly, one lone wave appeared and my friend, David Wilson, took off riding the wave perfectly all the way to the shore. His younger brother, Andrew, and I sat on our boards waiting for our rides, but no more waves appeared.

I remember distinctly wondering why the waves never seemed to show up explicitly for me. My insecurity surfaced, and

I was caught in a cycle of paranoid thoughts. *Then I looked around, took a deep breath, and accepted everything.* It was a spectacular scene we had paddled into. I suddenly felt totally connected, and right at that moment I looked over three dolphins swam out of the fog straight toward me. I was astounded as two of the dolphins passed close to me on each side, and the third dolphin in the middle, dove under the water, and swam right under me. He popped up on the other side, and the three dolphins swam away in perfect formation. And, right on cue, a flock of large pelicans flew very low, about fifteen feet directly over me. It was such an incredibly beautiful experience of perfect synchronicity and unity; I was left speechless. Andrew, who also witnessed the event was astounded too. We just sat there on our boards in the ocean, with our jaws dropped.

I don't remember catching even one wave that morning, but it didn't matter; it remains one of the most momentous surf sessions of my life.

Ceremony of the Sun

It was the rainy spring of 1998. Sheila, my wife, and I got married in Big Sur, California. It was a small, intimate, wedding ceremony consisting of only our immediate families. We stayed at the Ventana Inn, nestled in the beautiful hills overlooking the captivating California coastline and the Pacific ocean.

That spring had been the rainiest spring of the previous ten years. The winding mountain road leading to Big Sur had been closed for days due to rock slides. It finally opened the day before we were scheduled to be there, and we drove down the coast in the light rain from Monterey.

We had a beautiful dinner that night at the Inn. We woke up the next morning and prepared for our wedding ceremony. We had dreamed of having the wedding ceremony on Pfeiffer beach. However, it was still raining, and it looked like the ceremony would have to be held inside the Inn. I retreated to our cabin, nestled in the woods, to meditate in a big chair next to the open doors leading outside.

I remember distinctly letting go to God. I really wanted to get married on the beach, but whatever happened, I would be okay with it. I meditated for about twenty minutes. I opened my eyes as I came out of meditation, and right outside the glass doors leading into the woods – was a large wild turkey. I was amazed at how at ease the turkey was, being so close to me. Then out of the woods appeared a deer, who walked up right next to the turkey. Then a rabbit showed up, joining the turkey and the deer.

I looked at the wild animals, who were all so comfortable being so close to each other and to me, and I felt this intense sense of unity, and bliss. Sheila entered the room, and we watched the wild animals together, in awe.

We got dressed. We left the cabin. The rain had slowed to a light sprinkle, so we decided to head down to the beach. As we walked down the gentle path to the beach, the rain stopped completely, and just as we stepped onto the sand, the sun shined through a gap in the clouds. We were married on the beach in an incredibly beautiful ceremony with the waves crashing on the shore next to us.

Complete Acceptance

Accepting the present situation, accepting the Now, is hopefully illustrated in the stories above. It is a form of letting go, but there is a much deeper form of acceptance we also need to examine. It is complete acceptance. It feels like step seven, not step two because the concept is so profound, but here we go because without complete acceptance we really can't accept anything for very long.

Complete acceptance means you have to let go of who you think you are now. To be more specific, you have to let go of your

Step Two: ACCEPT

attachment to your temporary self that your mind has created. Your ego, which controls your mind, has done a very thorough job of creating the person you think you are; but unless you are totally awake, your idea of yourself is incomplete.

Everything in this life you create, including your body, your family, and your achievements, is temporary. It will all eventually turn back into dust. Yes, you can enjoy it while it lasts. Please do. However, you must eventually learn: *You must completely accept Being if you want eternal happiness.* The only way to experience that is to become aware of Being. In order to stay aware of Being, you need to accept completely. Complete acceptance is an essential step to enlightenment.

Maharishi used to tell a great story. Imagine you are living in a little wood hut with a dirt floor. You work hard to keep the little hut clean, and eventually, you put down a new wood floor to cover the dirt. You get new furniture, and the little hut is looking pretty good.

A King shows up and says; your hut is really nice, but he has a mind-blowing, marble palace near where you live, and he has business to take care of in the Far East. He won't be back for many years, maybe never, so you can live in his palace. He's always liked you. He'll give it to you. It's yours.

You look around at your little hut. You just got the new floor, and things are looking pretty good, so you decide to stay in the little hut because you can't believe the King would really give you his stunning palace anyway.

You are living in a small hut, but you can live in a monumental palace if you will just accept it. The little you, created by your ego, which you think is the only you, will never feel completely content or fulfilled. The big you, created by God, which is already surrounding you, is absolutely content, and totally fulfilled. You just have to become awake to the fact it is there, available to you at all times, and then accept the experience.

Forgiveness Allows Acceptance

Forgiveness is essential in life. Forgiveness is very powerful. Forgiveness allows acceptance. In order to truly accept someone you consider reprehensible, you have to forgive him or her first.

You also always need to forgive yourself. No matter what you did, no matter how deplorable you or others believe it is, you must totally forgive yourself. If you don't forgive yourself, your negative feelings will compound, and eventually, you will live an unhappy life that can even lead to sickness and death.

True forgiveness of others and yourself is letting go of your anger to the point of acceptance. Anything you completely accept, you will transcend. You will move beyond it.

Start off accepting the small irritations first, like the driver that races past you so fast on the highway you didn't even see him or her coming, and it startles you. I find it particularly obnoxious and also very dangerous, but if I am honest, I see exactly why that situation happens in my life.

As a teenager, I used to drive so fast, and recklessly, no one ever raced past me because I was racing past him or her. Then after a series of accidents, culminating in my near-death experience at Cornell, I finally learned to slow down and drive more responsibly. Now, the incredibly obnoxious driver I see in the rearview mirror, itching to speed past me, or the one that does race past, I try my very best to forgive him or her – because I realize it is what I have created; it is me. Our Higher Selves will always hold a mirror up to who we are so we can evolve past that hurdle. We attract in life what we are. We are all vibrating at specific, unique frequencies, and those frequencies will link up with similar frequencies. *What you like in others is what you like in yourself, and what you don't like in others is what you don't like in yourself.* Forgive others, and forgive yourself. Forgiveness allows acceptance. Acceptance allows transcendence. Transcendence is the key to experiencing Being.

Step Two: ACCEPT

Accept Evil to Eliminate Evil

When we encounter an evil situation in life, we should accept it, and then we should act to eliminate it. If our actions are not successful, we accept failure, and we continue to work to eliminate it. Always remember the first step to eliminating evil is to accept it.

As you become increasingly awake to the presence of Being, you will find you are living with less evil in your life, until you are actually living an extremely happy experience of Heaven on Earth. You may still witness evil from a distance, but it really won't be part of your life unless you let it.

This is not a selfish position. In fact, your deep awareness of Being will not only help you to achieve peace and happiness; it will help the entire world because ultimately we are all connected. When you change in a positive direction, you are helping everyone change in a positive direction. By naturally being your happy self, without any effort, you will elevate the vibration of others, and that will help them find happiness too.

Breathe Deeply and Accept

Acceptance of others negative behavior is not a mental position of spiritual superiority where you think to yourself; I will take the high road; this person is acting obnoxiously, but I will accept them. That is only a mental dialogue that will continue to perpetuate more anger. Total acceptance is where the attack has instigated a negative mental response, but you accept the situation, and your acceptance dissolves the anger. At first, this will take some practice, but eventually, as you are totally aware of Being, you will not be affected by the negative behavior of others for very long.

Practice acceptance. You are aware of the person behind you hitting their horn when you are too slow to take off after the light turned green. You start to become irritated, but you respond by taking a deep breath and accepting the situation. You naturally dissolve the anger, because you are not attached to it.

You are putting your attention, instead, on Being. Being is dissolving the anger. Being is allowing you to experience peace again. Don't fall into the trap of continuing a mental dialogue, attacking your attacker, or attacking yourself. Cut off the contentious mental dialogue by experiencing the peace of Being.

Practice acceptance, your experience will teach you it works. At first, your mind will automatically lead you into a defensive position. Your ego has trained you to defend it, and retaliate if necessary. Just witness your cycles of thinking and your increasing anger. As you witness and accept your own hostile thinking, it will transform into a positive position because you have become awake to a higher level of consciousness. *Your awareness of Being will automatically, effortlessly, dissolve the anger.*

Jesus said, "Judge not, that ye be not judged,"[4] not because there is some higher being in heaven called God that will dish out punishment if you judge. Jesus said that because when you judge someone, you are sending out negative energy, and negative energy automatically will attract negative energy back to you. Which is why he also said, "For with what judgment ye judge, ye shall be judged, and with what measure ye mete, it shall be measured to you again." [4] Not judging is acceptance.

You watch someone doing something you know is rude, or vulgar. Just accept them. They are being controlled by their rampant egos. Let it go. If they are sending negative energy into the Universe, they will reap what they have sowed; there is no need for you to defend yourself, or respond with your own attack. That will only include you in the creation of negative energy, and then you also will be creating a negative life for yourself.

If you can't shake the anger, and it starts to become a little monologue in your head, take a deep breath, take another, keep breathing until you break the chain of thinking – and then totally accept it. You may initially still be angry, fine, continue to accept it, then let it go. The key is not to attach yourself to the anger. The sooner you witness the anger and accept it, instead of attaching yourself to it, the better you will feel. You may have responded with harsh words or negative thoughts. Accept that too. Transcend it to experience Being.

Accept that You are in Control

The hard concept in life to understand, and then to always remember, is we are creating our own destiny every second of every minute, every hour of every day, every month of every year. *Our lives are completely our own creation.* We think and feel a certain way, and we believe life is this certain way, and that is exactly what we then experience. When you totally understand this to be true, it is incredibly freeing, and incredibly empowering.

We have no one else to blame in life – not our parents, not our ex-wife, or ex-husband, not our boss, not the government, not the president, or the rich 1%. Ultimately, none of them control our future – we do, and that is fantastic because now we can start living the way we want to live.

Sounds totally unrealistic, simplistic, and naive? You will just have to step back a few paces and watch the cause and effect relationship of what is going on in your life. You can also witness these laws of nature working with others, but be careful not to judge them. You know people in your life that always are victims. It is always someone else's fault. Their stories are very real, and, yes, in most cases, they have legitimate complaints about the way they have been treated in life, but why does life always pick on them? Why is their life always full of problems? Is it really just bad luck? No.

There is no such thing as bad luck or good luck. Your life is all created in exact accordance to what you project into the Universe. It is beyond total comprehension of how there are no accidents, and there is no randomness to any event, relationship, meeting, or creation. *We all, individually, as part of God, create every aspect of our own lives.*

The Universe Knows What You Want

Accept that the Universe already knows what you want. You have been sending out those desires for many years. *The Universe knows what you want and when you are awake to Being, if your desire is in accordance with Being, it will effortlessly appear in your life.* If your desire is not in accordance with Being, it may take longer, or it may never appear because your Higher Self knows you don't need it. You have reservations, doubts if it is right for you, and the Universe picks up on those doubts, so the signal sent into the Universe is not clear.

The irony of creation is that in order to reach the Source of all creation, Being, we need to transcend desires. Desires, and the cycle of thoughts they create keep us from experiencing Being. Stop thinking about your desires. The Universe already knows what you want. Transcend your desires. Accept the Now. When you start accepting and living in the Now on a regular basis, you will experience Being. The synchronicity of life will then amaze you as your desires begin to be created.

Ego Based Reality

Unfortunately, until you become aware of Being, your doubts and fears created by your ego-controlled mind, will appear as your reality. The anxiety, the mistakes, the bad luck, the sickness, even your own death is also created by you.

When I nearly died from my horrific car crash, I distinctly remember my last thoughts as my car flipped over twice, cartwheeling through the air, and it landed upside down, smashed into a telephone pole. I was feeling like there was some sort of major completion in that part of my life. I was done. I had just finished my last exam, my last lacrosse game, and I was ready for the summer; but overriding all of those thoughts was one *I actually felt*, one that was very powerful. It was a feeling of infinite power, and the desire to be so much more than I currently was.

I wanted to fly. I wanted to take off like Superman. I wanted enlightenment, but I didn't know how to recognize it yet. My Higher Self had to destroy my ego and who I thought I was first, and that is exactly what happened. This was my particular lesson. Our Higher Selves serve up lessons unique for each of us.

Our Higher Selves are always teaching us, guiding us to get back on the track to enlightenment in everything we do. The accident destroyed my ego, and it allowed me to become more aware of my Higher Self. Once I had briefly experienced higher consciousness, I wanted more. I wanted to be enlightened, and I have spent the rest of my life learning how to continually experience it. BANFEBA Meditation is the result.

Fantasy Life

Plan, and have goals in life. Choose your glorious path, but after the planning is done, don't let your mind drag you into a constant state of daydreaming about your fantasy future. *Always remember you have to transcend desires in order to experience the Source of creation, Being.* Don't continually feed your ego. Instead, slip back into acceptance, transcend thinking, become aware of Being, the feeling of Being, and you will become aware of how wonderful the life you are living is, right now. The irony is when you stop fantasizing about your goals, constantly chasing them, and you begin to accept the feeling you are living now, your goals will come to you faster because now you have the power of Being working for you.

Accept Your Prison of Fear in Order to Escape

Fear is a chain of thoughts that continues in cycles. Each thought is one of increased negativity. Fear is negative thought patterns that create negative energy. As the thoughts accumulate, fear takes over until the point it can become physically devastating. Sickness and disease is fear, negative thought patterns, that have rearranged the cells in your body in an unhealthy formation. Most people are able to check their fear, their negative energy, long enough to regain their health, but some don't, and eventually, death is the result.

Fear is our biggest enemy. As we get older, fear accumulates. We worry about our health. We worry about our bodies becoming frail and weak. We worry about our finances. We worry the ability to take care of our families. We worry about our jobs and the economy. The worries just go on and on, until we are living in a prison of fear.

The way to break free from fear is, to begin with a deep breath, then *accept* that the fear is present. Totally accept it. Feel it. Feel the fear and the doubt. Don't think about it. That will only feed it more. Just totally accept it, and allow the feeling to go inward, deeper. Your fear will naturally transform into the peaceful feeling of Being. Be aware of the absolute, silent, peaceful feeling of Being, and you are now free of fear. Being is the solution to all of your problems. So when you are experiencing Being, you are doing everything possible to be living a better, happier life.

You will actually feel the difference, and the feeling will give you the confidence you are on the right path. Continue the process of acceptance as much as possible in order to break the cycles of fear. Eventually, you will witness yourself slipping into a cycle of fear, and automatically you will be able to take a deep breath, accept, feel Being, and transcend the grip of fear. Acceptance is the key. *Acceptance allows you to become aware of Being. Acceptance is an essential step to enlightenment.*

Continual Acceptance Allows Continual Experience of Being

Continual acceptance in order to continually experience Being is a way of life. As you progress in your total understanding of the BANFEBA meditation technique, you will realize it is very simple. All Seven Steps merge into one step – *continual acceptance allows the continual experience of Being.*

Being is always there as the source of everything in creation at all times. When we don't experience Being, it is because we mistakenly identify with our ego. As soon as we accept the tangible feeling of Being, it is always there. We will begin to easily and effortlessly experience Being because it is our true nature. *We are expressions of Being.* We will naturally appreciate the experience of Being because it feels so peaceful, soothing, dynamic, and blissful.

The knowledge that has alluded many seekers of enlightenment, including me for so many years, is we don't have to go anywhere or do anything to experience Being. *We only have to accept Being, and it will appear.* Being is already here. On our spiritual paths, we are always implying we have to go to heaven to experience God. God is right here as the source of who we are. We only have to accept that to experience it. Always accept the tangible feeling of Being. Being is always here as the Source of us, and everything we experience in life. *Breathe and Accept the Now; Feel and Experience Being Awareness.*

Chapter Three

Step Three
NOW

Accept the Now

Another big misconception about enlightenment, which has confused many spiritual seekers, including myself for many years, is the belief that when you reach enlightenment, you will become someone else in your future that radiates a different state of consciousness. In fact, you don't become someone else, and nothing happens in the future. You are still you, and it all happens right now.

When you are enlightened, you are the same person with most of the same characteristics. Your experience of life, however, changes dramatically because of your awakening. Your ego still may influence your personality, but it will be in the background instead of leading you. You are led now by your Higher Self. You will now see the world in a totally new way, and that change in your perspective will influence major positive changes in your actual life.

Step Three: NOW

The transition doesn't happen in your future, it all happens right now. It is a very abstract concept, initially hard to comprehend, but through your experience of the Now, you will start to realize there is no future for *anything* to happen in. Life all happens now. *Everything that ever happens to you in your life is already a possibility at your Source, and it manifests, right now.* Life is digital, not analogue. It is like you are viewing a movie, projected digitally, not on actual film. You are attracting experiences to yourself, but your mind tricks you into believing there is a past, present, and future laid out in a timeline. Instead of projecting your life into a false future, transcend your desires, accept the Now. Experience the positive feeling of Being, right now.

Now is the Only Time You Can Experience Being

Accept the feeling you have right now. It doesn't matter what it is. It could be a feeling of fear, anxiety, frustration, jealousy or anger. Just feel it, deeply, now. *Breathe deeply, and accept the feeling you are having right now.* As you bring your awareness to the Now, without thinking, your experience of it will change, until you will feel Being as a deep, absolute peace in the background. Keep feeling the absolute peace of Being. Become aware that absolute peace is the Source of your reality.

Your experience transforms because the core of yourself, Being, is experienced as infinite peace. From this absolute, infinite, peaceful Being – happiness, love, and bliss will eventually blossom into your relative life. *Being, absolute peace, is the source of happiness, love, and bliss.* You must go to the Source, Being, first.

If you don't remain aware of Being, your current thought patterns become your current emotions and feelings. This is your ego. Your ego will inadvertently deceive you, and hide Being from you. Those thought patterns, driven by your ego, constantly reinforce an illusion of time with a past and a future. It makes it very hard to recognize; there is only the Now. As you practice BANFEBA, you will become awake to what is happening right now, and it will change your life in a very positive way.

Thinking about your past will not allow you to sustain happiness, daydreaming about your future will not allow you to sustain happiness; being present in the Now is the only way for you to sustain happiness. Once you have become awake to the Now and experienced this transformation, it will increase until the feeling of Being is automatic and instantaneous.

Use What is Happening Now to Experience Being

Listen to what is going on around you right now – the wind blowing, a plane flying overhead, a leaf blower in the neighbor's yard, the horns of cars stuck in traffic. Don't fight the sounds and wish to be in a quiet place to experience Being. Use the sounds, whatever they are, to bring yourself back to the present moment, back to the Now. Accept the sounds and listen without judging, then shift your awareness to the silence that surrounds the sounds. *Any sound presently occurring in your life, even an obnoxious sound, will take you to the Now, and the experience of Being if you accept it.*

Practice Being Aware of the Now

Like anything new in life, experiencing higher states of consciousness takes practice. The experience of Being is very subtle at first. It takes a lot of practice to allow that experience to become obvious to you. It takes a lot of repetition to automatically transcend thinking to become aware of the Now. It is a process of dismantling a lifetime of thinking. It takes time to re-identify. It takes time to totally understand you are not who you think you are; you are so much more.

Step Three: NOW

Live in the Now

What exactly is the Now? You may have heard various expressions describing experiencing the Now your whole life. Live in the Now. Be present. Let it Be. All of these expressions are saying the same thing – accept and experience the Now. The Now is the Absolute, the Source – God.

Zen Buddhism has trickled over from the East into our Western culture for centuries allowing us a glimpse into the philosophy of living in the Now. All other religions at their core speak of it too, sometimes using different terms. The contemporary version stripped of any confusing religious jargon is the brilliant book, *Power of Now*, by Eckhart Tolle. It is a clear explanation of being present in the Now. That precise knowledge works very well in conjunction with BANFEBA Meditation.

Different Paths to the Now

However, as brilliant and enlightened as Eckhart Tolle is, some people can't get past the first chapter of *Power of Now* before sliding it onto the shelf. I agree with every word of the book, but my wife, whom I love very much, and I consider very intelligent, and "awake," never finished it. At first, that bugged me. This is obviously the work of an enlightened master, how could she not see that?

Upon further contemplation I realized our Higher Self, Being, God, teaches us in every spiritual book every printed. We must pick one and study it, until we learn what it has to teach, and then find a new one that teaches us more. *The Bible* is one of the best spiritual books ever written. However, many people find it hard to decipher the Bible's archaic language, and its constant use of parables can be confusing. That does not discount the value of such books. They are still brilliant, and if we forced ourselves to study them, we would gain a lot, but gaining knowledge should not be hard. It should be easy.

The reason certain books click with some people, but not with others is that each book has a voice, and different voices resonate at different frequencies. Find a frequency that matches your own, then the knowledge contained within will be easy for you to digest. We can't rely on only one book or one teacher to teach all of humanity. Life is not that simple.

We each have our own unique and valid spiritual paths in life. We must respect our paths and everyone else's path. We may think some of those paths, others choose, are not overtly "spiritual." It doesn't matter what we think. Those paths are absolutely perfect for those people, at those particular stages of their lives. We may not be able to recognize it, but there is no need to – just accept it.

The Art of Now

What is the Now? The Now is everything that is happening exactly, precisely, right now. When I was 16, I was studying photography at Andover, and I was introduced to the work of Henri-Cartier Bresson. I believe, in retrospect, Henri-Cartier Bresson was the most influential artist in my life. My initial work in photography was the catalyst that eventually led me to filmmaking.

Henri-Cartier Bresson could display an entire movie in one single frame.

Bresson's photography instantly resonated with me in such an impactful way. I didn't know it at the time, but I was already searching for experiences of the Now, and Bresson spent his entire life searching for images that expressed, "*The Decisive Moment.*" When Bresson first saw a photograph by Hungarian photographer, Martin Munkacsi, titled *Three Boys at Lake Tanganyika*, he said, "I suddenly understood that a photograph could fix eternity in an instant."[5] Bresson's genius was in allowing the dynamic, profound unity of the present moment to be expressed in his photographs.

Step Three: NOW

My goal as an artist in this lifetime is to be able to express the dynamic, profound unity of the present moment in an entire feature film. I want to capture, and express twenty-four frames a second for two hours of "decisive moments." The only way to create on such a transcendental level is to continually, totally accept, and live in the Now. Art always reflects the consciousness of the artist.

Extreme Experience of the Now

What is the Now? The Now is the razor-sharp second happening exactly right now. You can experience the Now, only if you can transcend your thinking. You have felt the Now many times in your life, even if you are not completely aware of it, but the experiences were most likely fleeting because your thinking mind hides the experience from you.

What is the tangible, real feeling of the Now? The experience of the Now at the surface level is as varied and as infinite as the Universe we live in, but there are common experiences at the core – a deep silence, profound feeling of peace, and absolute interconnectedness with everything and everyone you encounter. BANFEBA Meditation technique will allow you to experience the Now on a regular basis, but for reference, there are other examples of life experiences that sometimes give the same result, temporarily.

When you have an *extreme experience,* you slip into the Now. Everything slows down, and you are completely aware, in extraordinary detail, of what is happening right now. In sports, people call this entering "The Zone," mentioned earlier. One way we slip into the Zone is through an extreme experience.

One day, many years ago, I went bungee jumping with a friend. We hiked into the mountains outside of Los Angeles with a group of about ten people. About two hours into the mountains, we ran into an abandoned single span bridge built in 1936. The road leading to it was washed out in a giant flood, so the bridge remained in the mountains, alone, with no roads leading to it. It is commonly referred to as, "The Bridge to Nowhere."

We climbed out onto the center of the bridge and looked down a hundred feet below to the rocky stream. I watched a few others tying off a long bungee cord to the bridge and the other end to a metal brace on their ankles. They took turns standing on top of the railing and diving out into free fall.

Bungee-jumping is unnerving to even watch, and it is totally petrifying to partake in. When I was a young boy, I was actually afraid of heights, and I had to conquer my fear to even climb a tall ladder, or stand on a roof, but throughout my life, I made it one of my missions to never let fear control me.

I dove out in a swan position, and I dropped a hundred feet below. I watched the walls of the cliff on either side of the bridge drop away, giving a pronounced feeling of speed as I fell. Then everything felt like it was in slow motion. I reached the bottom, coming dangerously close to the boulders in the stream below. The thick elastic bungee cord whipped me back into the air, and I flew back up, a hundred feet, almost hitting the bridge above. Then down again, back up, and down. I eventually settled, and they pulled me up to the bridge. When I finally reached safety, the adrenaline was still speeding through my body so fast I felt higher than a kite. As it dissipated, I wanted more.

After that extreme experience, I got heavily addicted for a couple of years to the sport of hang gliding for the same reason. Each weekend, I would stand on the top of a three thousand foot mountain, and I would jump off with a wing on my back. I would fly over the mountains like a bird. After I landed I felt so high; it lasted for days. Later in the week, I wanted more so, I went out that weekend, and I jumped off the mountain again. I repeated that cycle for two years, until I crashed badly, broke my

Step Three: NOW

ankle in three places, and my wife, Sheila, told me if we wanted to have a child, I would have to give up hang gliding because it was too dangerous. I agreed, it wasn't worth the risk, so I quit flying. I had gone way beyond my mission of conquering fear – now I was actually seeking it out.

Looking back at the experience I know exactly why it was so incredibly addicting. It was not only the surge of adrenaline. It was an example of an extreme experience. It was a forced entry into the Now whether you wanted to go or not. The experience is so intense and so precarious, you can't be aware of anything else except what is happening exactly right now.

Besides bungee jumping and hang gliding, I have experienced that same feeling heli-skiing in Canada, mountain climbing in Wyoming, and surfing big waves in Malibu. It is a sensational feeling, and those are some of the best experiences of my life, but truthfully, any experience, extreme or gentle, that allows you to become awake to the present moment will open the doorway to the Now.

When my son, Weston, who I love so incredibly much, was thirteen years old, he loved the super scary roller coasters at Magic Mountain amusement park in Los Angeles. I was his riding partner. At that stage in my life, a walk across the parking lot could thrill me, so I didn't necessarily need to be shot a hundred feet into the air like a rocket or tossed in circles like a sneaker in a clothes dryer, but Weston absolutely loved it, so off I'd go. Just being in his presence is a constant source of joy for me.

As I watched him next to me on a thrilling ride, I knew why he and countless others are addicted to roller coasters, paintball, mountain biking, kite-surfing, base-jumping, or countless other "extreme sports." They are being catapulted into the present moment, and once they have experienced it, they want more. It is like being addicted to heroin or cocaine. It feels great, but like being addicted to a drug, the ending isn't always good for those addicted to extreme experiences. A life-threatening situation does have the ability to push you into the Now, but I don't recommend using it as a technique to become enlightened. It can also kill you.

The handsome actor, and star of the *Fast and Furious* movies, Paul Walker, was killed in a horrific car crash. He was the passenger in a Porsche going way too fast. He, like the legendary actor, James Dean, many years before, was addicted to the thrill induced by speed, and his life was sadly, cut terribly short. I felt empathy for them both because I knew exactly what pushed them to go so fast.

When I was at Cornell the year before my near fatal car crash, I drove up to Watkins Glenn, New York in 1978, where they held the US Grand Prix from 1961-1980. I was thrilled to photograph the Formula One drivers racing incredibly fast on the winding track. The adrenaline was contagious. Soon, a few of my crazy friends and I all wanted to be race car drivers, and we would recklessly street race whenever we got a chance.

Now it is easy for me to trace back further in my life to see where this seed was planted, and how life is all interconnected. When I was eight years old in 1966, the first movie I ever saw on the big screen was John Frankenheimer's epic, *Grand Prix*. On a rainy afternoon, my dad dropped my two brothers and me off at the theatre to watch the movie. When the MGM Lion growled at the start of the movie it was so loud my younger brother, Hunt, who was only six years old, started crying, and my older brother, John, who was ten, had to sit in the lobby with him because Hunt didn't dare enter the theater. I watched the movie with great excitement, alone, glued to my seat, and it made an indelible impression on me.

When I recently saw Ron Howard's movie, *Rush*, and saw the scene where racing legend, Niki Lauda, was horrifically

Step Three: NOW

burned in a bad crash, it brought back a distinctive memory. I was at the US Grand Prix, in Watkins Glenn in 1978, standing near the pit crew, photographing the drivers entering their cars. I noticed one cool-looking Austrian driver, Niki Lauda, pick up his helmet and face mask, but before slipping the mask over his head, he turned, and I noticed the whole opposite side of his face was completely destroyed by scar tissue from a horrific crash two years earlier.

If I had been more aware, it could have been a warning sign for me to recognize, but I was young, naive, and I had been blinded by my fantasy of Formula One race car driving. I was too busy watching the beautiful girls swarm around the dashing Formula One champion, Niki Lauda's nemesis – James Hunt.

My near-death car crash at Cornell the next year was the worst and last of four major car accidents I was involved in. I was only driving in two of those accidents, my crazy friends were driving in the other two, but the addiction to speed during an extreme experience was involved in all four accidents. I was a slow learner, and like a fool, I didn't realize the consequences of my addiction. It was only by nearly killing a friend I learned to quit. He too was addicted to speed and loved to race with me, but if he is going to die, let it be his own foolish driving that kills him, not mine.

Extreme experiences will push the limits of whom we are in order to reach for more because innately we all know there is so much more out there for us to experience. During the mid-eighties, when I was trying to launch my first movie, *Real Cowboy*, my film editor, Larry, introduced me to a good friend of his, Anne, who introduced me to her very close friend, Bob Weir, from the Grateful Dead band. I was always a big fan of their music, but my incentive in meeting Bob was to try to convince him to join the cast of my first movie so all of his devoted "Deadhead" fans would see it.

I was a lot younger than Bob, but we got along brilliantly, sitting up all night on a few occasions, philosophizing on the meaning of life. At that point, I was mostly done with experimenting with drugs, because I was concentrating so much on meditation, but Bob taught me something that still sticks with me today. Bob believed so many rock stars were addicted to drugs because the feeling of being on stage in front of thousands of adoring fans was such an adrenaline-inducing high when you stepped backstage, and it was over, you desperately wanted more, and drugs, as dangerous as they are, got you there.

During one of his big concerts in upstate New York, I hung out on stage hiding behind one of the gigantic speakers, and I got a small taste of what Bob Weir, Jerry Garcia, and all other rock stars experience regularly. It is staggering to look out at a sea of people all looking back at you with such love in their eyes. It is an extreme experience. It is an experience of the Now.

My father in law, Fred, was a Marine during the Viet Nam War. He was wounded in battle during the Tet Offensive in 1968, and he received the Bronze Star for bravery. We both love movies, and we have had many long discussions about all movies, but I always specifically quiz him about what it was like during the war, and what war movies are the most real. Through that process, one comment he once made has always stuck with me. He explained that some soldiers, don't talk about it much, but for them, combat is extremely exciting, and it can become addicting. Like drugs and extreme sports, war can be addictive, because you are having an extreme experience.

After the initial pain – death ends up being the complete extreme experience. I already told you of my near-death experience, but I also know from other experiences, even being near death can give you the experience of the Now.

When I was studying filmmaking at Columbia University in New York City, I remember one cold, rainy, winter afternoon.

Step Three: NOW

I was walking fast on Broadway trying to enter the subway at 86th Street to get up to Columbia for a meeting with my screenwriting professor to discuss my first feature film script he had just read.

I was excited and moving fast. It was raining hard, and my eyes were focused on the large puddles I was trying to avoid when for some reason I looked up to my right, and I saw a frail old lady, who must've been about eighty-five. She was still trying to walk with her cane across Broadway, but the light had already changed to green, and cars were now racing past her. I looked up from the puddles just as a large truck, barreling down Broadway, switched lanes, and ran her over without even stopping.

Everything went into slow motion as I watched her get run over by the massive back wheels. I could even clearly see the horrific expression on her face, and hear her gasp. The driver didn't even see her. He must've thought he hit a pothole when the rear tires bumped into the air as he drove over her body because he just kept going.

I immediately ran out into the street to help, extending my hand, trying to stop traffic from doing any further damage, but when I looked to my feet at her body, and I saw her head completely crushed, and her brains literally splattered onto the pavement, it was obvious there was no saving her.

A police officer, a street patrolman, ran out into the street after me. He saw her brains steaming from the heat on the cold rainy street, took his jacket off, and threw it onto her. His partner joined us and replaced me to stop traffic. The first cop flagged down a car to chase after the fleeing truck.

I got to my meeting with my screenwriting professor, and I started to tell him the story. He stopped me as I got to the description of the steaming brains on the street, and he muttered he couldn't hear any more. I didn't want to act ghoulish, but the truth is my own personal feeling was one of peace. I felt the old lady was in a good place now. It may have been a tough trip to heaven, but I knew she was okay.

For more than twenty years, as a volunteer, I have mentored at-risk youth in Watts, Los Angeles. The housing project, Nickerson Gardens, and the surrounding area where the kids live has one of the highest homicide rates in the country. During the nineties, when I was mentoring there a couple days a week, it was like the wild west; bullets were flying, and you could constantly hear police helicopters flying overhead trying to track down the shooters.

Once, when I was coaching baseball to a team of Latino and African American kids from the neighborhood in the Ted Watkins park close to Nickerson Gardens, I was standing at home plate, hitting balls to the players in the field. Out of the corner of my eye, I saw a young teenager, about sixteen, riding a bike past another who was walking. As he rode past, he pulled out a 38 mm pistol, and he shot him, point blank, right in the chest. The second boy flew back onto the ground. I dropped my bat, raced around the backstop to help, and as I ran past the shooter, who was still holding the gun only a few feet away, everything went into slow motion. The kid just looked at me, laughed like it was all a big game, and he rode off.

I dropped to my knees next to the boy who was bleeding profusely from a large hole in his chest, and I grabbed his hand. I talked to him, trying to calm him, trying to let him know everything was going to be all right. A distraught lady, a mother from the neighborhood, was screaming manically for the constant violence she had witnessed too many times, to stop killing their babies. An ambulance, two squad cars, and a police helicopter flying overhead, all arrived immediately.

I ended up writing an antagonistic letter to the mayor of Los Angeles, fighting for more government-sponsored mentoring programs to stop the gang violence, and my story was later printed in the Los Angeles Times, but in that exact moment, the truth was, everything was okay.

Life is precious, and we should work to preserve it in any way we can. Gang violence has to stop, and I have worked for years to help stop it, but the actual experience of death, once the initial pain of the dying body has passed, is extremely pleasant.

Both of my parents have now died, and I was standing right beside each of them when they passed away. It was a very emotional experience losing someone I loved so much, and I cried profusely, but the truth is deep inside, once I let the drama of my thoughts subside, and I accepted it, I felt okay. We always want to cherish and respect life. We want to fight to the end to stay alive, but when death does come, it is a profound awareness of Being, God, and we all will be fine.

Become Awake to the Now

In retrospect, I realize relying on extreme experiences to help us become awake to the Now is actually tantamount to insanity. I hope my son, Weston, is evolved enough to skip that sophomoric stage of testosterone driven machismo. Not only is it destructive, and life-threatening, but it is not a successful method of stabilizing your life in the Now. It will always only be a temporary experience.

Instead of fighting your fear head on, it is much smarter to transcend your fear. *Accept your fear to transcend your fear.* Fighting your fear is only your ego fighting your ego. Once you have conquered your fear, your ego can brag about it, but it is a never-ending cycle, and in the end, death is the only winner.

Our experience doesn't have to be terrifying or death-defying for us to become awake to the Now. When you slip into a hot Jacuzzi, or a warm bath on a cold winter day after working or playing outside, the soothing feeling of the hot water allows you to briefly transcend your thinking mind. It is such an absolutely calming feeling you are easily able to transcend your thinking. All of your senses are overwhelmed by the feeling of hot water against your body. That also can be an experience of the Now. You are able to transcend your desires because in that exact moment you are so content you desire nothing else.

When you make love, and reach orgasm, that too is a taste of the present moment. When you share a deep laugh with someone you love or even a stranger, that is a brief experience of the Now. When you sit in silence and watch a snowflake fall from the sky, and it is so beautiful you can think of nothing else. That is an experience of presence. Presence is the Now. It is always there. We only have to become awake to it.

Living in the Now is a Sublime Experience

The vehicle to become present in the Now does not have to be sensual, romantic, visually enticing, or induced by some life-threatening act. Living in the Now is a truly sublime connection with everything in existence that allows your experience of living to become more profound and enjoyable.

Just as there are many frequencies of sound comprised to make up one song, there are many different relative experiences created from the Now. Conversely, these experiences can all be used to link up with the Now, which at its core is absolute, infinite, peaceful, silence.

The key is not to try to totally, completely, understand it, because no human ever totally will. Even if you are enlightened, you never will understand it because the Now is the Source of all creation, and it is infinite. Infinity cannot be completely understood, or it would be finite. You will understand more and more at each new level of awareness, but your understanding will always continue to evolve because the knowledge is infinite. Just experience Being, the Now, become awake to it and enjoy it. Remember, life is eternal, enjoy each new experience, and each new level of awareness.

Step Three: NOW

Create Now

If you have read any of the books on "The Law of Attraction," and you are still not rich yet, it is because the only place and time that allows what you want to be created are here in the Now. The more you chase your specific desires, dreaming about them, hoping to attract them, the further they will be from becoming your reality because your fantasy is pushing them into a fictitious future. You must transcend your desires to be present in the Now. Now is where everything is created.

The Law of Attraction sounds so simple. It's not. If it were, everybody who ever read those books would be extremely rich and successful. The basic principals behind The Law of Attraction are true. But it is impossible to manipulate the Source. You can only accept success through The Law of Attraction. And you can only accept success in the Now. Once you start to experience Being on a regular basis, you will begin to get what you need. You will become happy, healthy, prosperous, and fulfilled. The trick to creating those desires is to transcend the desires. The desires are keeping you from experiencing Being where complete fulfillment is experienced.

Right Now, Your World is Your Creation

The fundamental principals of The Law of Attraction that validate it surround you. Right now – your car, your clothes, your house, your spouse, your child, parents, friends, partner, job, boss – everything in your world down to the last detail is your creation. *Your thoughts lead to feelings, which create your reality.* They continuously create the world you presently live in. Put it to the test – look at your own life, everything in it, at one point was a desire, an impulse, or a fear.

Your life is your movie. You are the writer, director, and star. Your thoughts, feelings, and emotions are the film going through the projector. You are projecting the images of your life onto the screen. The life you are currently living is the story on the screen. You can change your life in any way you want if you change your thoughts and feelings accordingly. However, changing your thoughts and feelings is not as easy as it seems. You need to be experiencing the Source, Being, first. Transcend your desires. This will allow you to experience Being, then the life you wish to live will effortlessly appear.

The Buzz

In the late eighties when I was spending a lot of time at meditation retreats, I once had a miraculous experience that illuminated the mechanics of our ability to create our own lives, clearly to me.

I was sitting in lotus position, on a pillow, on the floor of a room, alone, in an old Victorian house in Connecticut. I had been meditating for hours. It was my second day of extended meditation. Suddenly, I was very much aware of a big black fly, buzzing loudly, in the room. I opened my eyes and watched him cruise around the room. He was a large black fly that sounded like a loud, mini crop-dusting plane. I looked around the room, wondering how this noisy invader had entered my peaceful space. The large windows were closed, and the door to the hallway was closed. Had he been sleeping for hours, and he suddenly awoke to ruin my meditation? The vision of me chasing the fly around the room to swat him, so I could get back to my meditation, didn't feel exactly right. Somehow, I felt connected to the little guy. In fact, as I accepted the situation, and I began to effortlessly allow him to fly noisily around the room, I felt totally at one with him. Then I noticed a light, coming from the hallway, shining through the gap at the bottom of the door. I wondered if the fly had entered the room by flying under the door? I had never seen that happen before, but maybe he did.

I became slightly excited, while still meditating, peacefully witnessing this big black fly buzzing around the room. I had

Step Three: NOW

the desire to see if I could get the fly to actually fly back out under the door, and leave me in peace. Sounds impossible? Communicating with a fly? But that is exactly what I did.

I effortlessly had the thought, and I visualized the flight pattern. I had the desire, and then I let it go. I transcended all desires. I remained very present, without any expectations, and sure enough, the big black fly, flew down, right out under the door. At the time, it felt strangely normal. Now looking back on it, it was a total miracle. Did I actually talk to a fly and tell him to fly under a door? Did he comply with my request and pull off a move that is very strange indeed? Well, yes, and no. I did ask, but I also complied. I became one with the Source, the core of everything in Universe, and so it was merely an extension of myself that flew under the door. It is not exactly the most glorious example of creating one's destiny, but it was extremely enlightening for me.

Most of our big desires remain unfulfilled until we spend years working hard to achieve them, and even then, many desires seem unobtainable because we don't go to the Source first. However, as you become more awake, you will start to notice your little desires are being created for you all of the time because you are not obsessed with them. You are not thinking about them constantly. You are letting them go. You are transcending your desire.

It is a cloudy Sunday afternoon, and you're watching a baseball game or a movie on TV, and suddenly you have a strong desire for something sweet. You want some candy, cookies, or ice cream, but you don't feel like getting in your car and traveling to the store, so you let it go, and you settle back into your chair to finish watching the movie or game. A few minutes later the doorbell rings, and you open the door to discover a Girl Scout is selling cookies. Perfect! You love the chocolate mint cookies, and you buy two boxes. As you settle back, eating the delicious cookies, if you are awake, you will realize a miracle just happened.

The Red Sea did not part, but still, the odds of the cookies showing up at just that time are so far beyond any type of normal logic it can only be explained as a small miracle. That type of creating happens on a daily basis if you look at your life carefully.

Of course, if you are all stressed out, anxious, and irritable with negative feelings and emotions, then that negative world becomes your creation too. The Girl Scout doesn't show up. Instead, you get the guys selling magazines you don't want, and it further irritates you they are allowed to invade your space to sell you things. That leads to more negative thoughts about the abuse of our space by advertisers, etc., and you've had these thoughts before, and everywhere you look you see more advertising, and oh it feels so unnatural to you – billboards, TV ads, posters, Internet spam, texts! Advertising is like a plague. You wonder how did we go so far in this direction? We created it, that's how. And the more you think it bugs you, the more it will. The more you hate anything in life, the more you will see it arrive at your doorstep. If you despise a certain racial profile because of some lingering prejudice you inherited from your parents during your childhood, guess who is going to move into the house across the street that was just put up for sale? Look closely at your life. It happens continuously. Each of us, create our own unique existence down to the last detail.

So why don't we just meditate, slip into the Now, and totally believe our lives have no bugs, no unwanted advertising, and are full of Girl Scouts hand delivering our favorite cookies? Well, yes: we can create those things in our lives. Can we create a million dollars? Definitely. Is it harder? Yes. When we get to Chapter Nine, we will discuss the mechanics of creation in more detail.

Listen to the Song of Life

Listening can be another vehicle to the Now. That happy feeling you experience when a good song comes on the radio is you slipping into the Now, because your listening has become so focused, you are just feeling, not thinking. When you dance, you listen in order to respond to the music, and listening innocently allows you to slide into the Now.

One of the very best acting teachers, Sanford Meisner, working out of the Neighborhood Playhouse in New York City from the 50's – 90's developed an extraordinary acting technique many of Hollywood's stars still use today called the Meisner Technique, based on listening. When an actor is actively listening, he or she cannot be thinking, and the response will be more real because the self-conscious thinking will have been transcended. If you want help winning an Academy Award for acting, slip into the Now. God is an excellent actor.

Cycles of Thought Keep Us From the Now

Most of the thoughts we have today are tantamount to the thoughts we had yesterday. We think in cycles, and those patterns of thinking can be carried through an entire lifetime. Most of these thought cycles are driven by incessant desires we perpetually have. Your thought cycles block you from fully experiencing the Now. In Sanskrit, those cycles or patterns of thoughts are called "Pragyapradh," which loosely translated means "mistake of the intellect." It is a mistake because the intellect thinks those cycles of thoughts are who it is. Your thoughts are not who you are. They are merely fleeting impressions passing through. Don't become attached to them. Don't judge yourself based on your thoughts. Don't become your thoughts. Transcend your thoughts, and return to the Now.

Return Home

Eventually, after practicing BANFEBA, you will be able to return to the Now at command, and it will be incredibly liberating. When you catch yourself thinking in a cycle of negative thoughts, or a pattern of fantasies, and then you return to the Now, it will be like returning home, and it will feel soothing, and comfortable. *The profound feeling of Being is so peaceful; it feels so innately natural because it is who you really are.*

Fresh Start Now

Your thoughts are very good at trapping you, keeping you from experiencing Being. It always seems so important to figure out through extensive thinking a solution to your problems in order to take the best step forward. The irony is your thoughts are what is keeping you attached to your problems.

The thoughts are totally binding if something really despicable has happened to you recently, but sometimes the cycles of thought can be traced all the way back to your childhood. A lot of the time, your troubled past continues to irritate you, and influence your current moods. Whether your thoughts are traced back to a continuous loop you have experienced since your childhood, or whether they are related to some current drama you are presently living, the result is the same – your thoughts are trapping you – keeping you from experiencing Being.

The most important thing to remember is you can always have a fresh start, a new beginning to your life, right now. When you become awake to the Now, and experience Being, you are brand new. That is true forgiveness. That is what Jesus was really teaching. God, Being, always completely forgives you, right now.

You don't have to follow some archaic ritual of chanting, prayer, or repenting, to be forgiven. Follow the Seven Steps, and when you experience the absolute silence and peace of Being, it will all make complete sense. Let your experience be your teacher. *Breathe and Accept the Now; Feel and Experience Being Awareness.*

Chapter Four

Step Four
FEEL

Feel Being

You can experience Being through all five of the senses – seeing, tasting, smelling, hearing, and feeling. As you become more awake, you will notice expanded awareness is achieved through each of the senses. This is good. Keep using all five senses to experience Being. However, with the BANFEBA Meditation technique Feeling is the initial sense used because you can use your entire body to feel. It is a tangible experience that is easy to recognize, and good to begin with.

    Left alone in life, we will naturally gravitate towards whatever feels better. Watch yourself – you're cold; you put on a sweater or turn up the heat. You're thirsty; you drink. You're hungry; you eat. You're lonely; you call a friend. Even on a more subtle level it is still true. Without thinking, we will turn our gaze from the ugly trash in the gutter to the beautiful sunset. Someone is laughing;

we unconsciously will turn and listen. Someone smiles at you; you like it, and automatically smile back. Young lovers embrace; we look. An old lady and man hold hands; innately, we like it. A beautiful person walks into the room – we will appreciate the beauty. Someone shows us compassion or true love for any reason, and we appreciate it. Why, do we respond this way? Because, it feels good, and it leads us back to whom we really are – we are innately a positive expression of Being. The course of our lives will always naturally lead us back to whom we are.

Feeling good is contagious. We project what we think and feel, as vibrations, into our immediate environment, and it continues out into the Universe. Those positive feeling vibrations link up with other positive feeling vibrations and are attracted back to us.

Feeling at peace is our natural state. The feeling of deep peace is the state of Being at our very core, and if we can transcend our continuous thought patterns, we will automatically gravitate to the peaceful feeling of Being. We create negativity in our lives through negative thoughts perpetuated by our ego. Negativity links up with more negativity, and soon that becomes our reality. However, always remember to use negativity as a road sign to direct us back to Being.

At our core is Being. Being is the absolute Source where everything that is good, pure, beautiful, happy, peaceful, and loving, expresses itself in the relative world we live in. Being is our natural state hidden by our thinking. We experience Being by transcending thinking. It is a state of awareness where thinking may accompany it in the background, but it is not attached to it.

When we see the beautiful, innocent child laugh, we laugh or smile too. At first, we don't think, we just laugh or smile. We might then think, wow, what a cute child, but the thought is secondary and really unnecessary. The happy feeling will come without the thought. The thought did not make us happy. The child's energy of love we linked up with did.

Negative Feelings are Indicators to Get You Back on Track

You are waiting in line at the bookstore. It is Christmas time, the place is packed, and the line is long. People are rushing to buy books to complete their gift list. You are stuck in the long line, you have lots to accomplish today, and you feel anxious. Take a deep breath, take another, accept the situation now, take another breath, and feel Being. Wow, feel the excitement in the air. The line is moving. Take another deep breath, accept the Now, transcend your desire to move faster, transcend thinking, feel, and experience Being. Wow, you are feeling better. You look around; you're next in line. The line moved fast, and now people seem happy. You're happy.

Feel Your New World

What just happened? What happened is you just changed your world. You changed, and the world, which is a reflection of you, changed too. Try it, and let your experience teach you it is true.

The Art of Science

When I was studying color photography at Cornell, I used to search all over campus for vibrant colors to shoot; then I would spend hours in the darkroom, trying to bring them to life.

One special day, I found this big open field on the edge of campus. My eye located a massive, bright orange, industrial-sized, metal container on a hill overlooking the field. I climbed the hill and shot some great abstract photographs of the container. The photographs ended up earning me a lot of acclaim from my photography professor, who told me I should definitely continue exploring photography. I had no idea what I was shooting that day – I was led by my intuition. Upon reflection, I saw significance in what I had created, and it became a theme I worked with for years; there is art in absolutely everything.

I discovered later, the bright orange canister was part of an Electron-Positron Collider, which is a very expensive, elaborate, enormous contraption built under the field that accelerates then collides atoms with the goal of trying to find smaller, and smaller particles of matter, in order to ultimately discover what is at the Source of life, as we know it. Cornell University had recently built one on campus. When I discovered the field in 1979, it was brand new.

I am not a scientist, but I believe those expensive particle accelerators will never ultimately discover exactly what the Source is because the Source of creation is beyond matter. The Source is the nothingness behind the something. It is the space between things, but it is nothing. It is the Source of the sound vibration, but it is not sound. The Source is infinite, and beyond total comprehension, but you can still experience it. That is the key, experience it, feel it, and create with a connection to it, but don't try to completely understand it, because you never totally will.

Max Planck, a German theoretical physicist, who originated quantum theory, and won the Nobel Prize in Physics in 1918, summed it up perfectly, "Science cannot solve the ultimate mystery of nature, and that is because, in the last analysis, we ourselves are part of the mystery that we are trying to solve."[6] Albert Einstein also figured it out many years ago – "Anyone who is seriously involved in the pursuit of science becomes convinced that a spirit is manifest in the laws of Universe – a spirit vastly superior to that of man."[7]

Practice Feeling Being

The more you are able to feel Being, the more you will become awake to it, and the more you will experience it. You will eventually reach the stage where it becomes automatic. You are aware of a stressful situation, you breathe deeply, accepting the

Now, and you feel the stress release. The stress completely fades away. You feel peaceful and happier. Happiness attracts more happiness, and it becomes the state of consciousness you are now experiencing.

You have felt higher states of consciousness before, and you will naturally gravitate towards that if you give yourself the opportunity. Through the Seven Steps, you naturally are able to experience it. Practice feeling it.

Mantra Meditation

Meditation using a mantra (from the Vedic tradition) is also one of the best methods of transcending thinking to experience the feeling of Being. The Transcendental Meditation technique is one of the best Vedic mantra meditation techniques taught by qualified teachers. Transcendental Meditation uses a mantra, which is a Sanskrit word given to you by a trained TM teacher. Mantras have been used in Vedic meditation techniques taught by Hindu and Buddhist monks and gurus for many centuries.

You can read about mantras and their different effects in several great books by a contemporary Vedic scholar named Thomas Ashley-Farrand. However, mantra meditation can be very powerful, and if used without the proper instruction, it can have adverse effects. If you are interested in further exploration of meditation techniques using a mantra, you should either take the TM course or be taught by another qualified teacher. You could go online, and get a mantra, but you'll probably end up with a lot of headaches, and it could take your whole life before you figure it out. Proper practice of meditation is a specific process that needs guidance. If you want to meditate using a mantra properly, find a qualified teacher.

A mantra is a Sanskrit word, but like all words, it vibrates at a certain sound frequency. When you think the mantra, effortlessly, to yourself, and thinking it effortlessly is the key, that mantra, because it is vibrating at a specific frequency, allows you to transcend thinking to experience higher states of consciousness. If you are presently practicing TM or another Vedic mantra meditation technique, please continue. If you supplement the mantra technique with the Seven Steps, you can expedite your awakening dramatically. You will be experiencing Being at all times not only when you are meditating using a mantra. BANFEBA is something you can do all day long, every day, and it becomes a habit in the way you live your life. The results become much more powerful and dynamic.

Yoga

Yoga has become extremely popular in America. Where I live in Santa Monica, California, every day I see people walking, riding bikes, skateboarding, and driving to yoga classes carrying their rolled-up yoga mats. This yoga crowd, in many instances, started practicing yoga to get in shape physically, and for that purpose, yoga works very well.

Yoga also helps you stay agile, and coordinated. I have played sports my entire life, and I have had many sports-related injuries with broken bones, torn ligaments, tendons, etc. Those accidents tend to catch up to you when you get older, but because I practice yoga each day, my body still feels great, and I am limber enough to skateboard around Santa Monica with my 15-year-old son, Weston.

Most people practicing yoga extensively have discovered yoga is much deeper than just getting in shape or staying limber. Yoga is thousands of years old, from the discipline of Ayurveda. In the ancient Vedic language, Sanskrit, yoga means a union of spirit and body. Yoga is a technique to help you reach higher states of consciousness, and it works very well in conjunction with meditation.

Step Four: FEEL

Yoga is extremely beneficial in allowing you to actually feel the subtle energy of Being flowing in your body effortlessly. You should learn simple yoga postures, "Asanas," and practice them privately each day. It only takes about 10 minutes. If you also want to supplement your private practice with yoga classes, that is also beneficial.

Thoughts are not Feelings

It is imperative to distinguish between thoughts and feelings. Thoughts and feelings are interrelated, but there is a distinction, and it is good to experience the distinction. Thinking and feeling are linked but still separate.

If you are having angry thoughts, you can begin to feel anxious and upset because you are resisting Being in the background. You are not accepting the Now. Your awareness is becoming clouded over. You have lost awareness of Being. Those negative physical feelings will compound as they link up to similar feelings. Eventually, you can even become sick. You can break the negative cycle and heal yourself if you become aware of and feel Being. Being is the source of perfect health.

Breathe deeply, and accept what you are feeling now. You may become aware of your negative thinking as if it is a radio or a TV playing in the background. Don't contribute to the cycle of thinking, just accept your thinking. Take another deep breath; accept your current feeling, innocently, effortlessly feel it, and it will transform into the peace of Being.

Thoughts are precursors to feelings. Thinking positive, therefore, can help lead to feeling healthy and happy; however, it is almost impossible to instantly change your course of thinking from negative to positive. We always hear the refrain: think positive! But, when you are mad, it is very hard to immediately switch your thought pattern. The key is not to fight the thinking and forcefully try to stop negative thoughts but to transcend the negative thinking. Feel whatever is presently there, and accept it. It will naturally transform into what is always subtly there in the background – Being.

Being will feel peaceful, and that wonderful feeling of deep peace will link to more positive feelings. Take a deep breath, accept the current good feeling, innocently stay aware of it, and enjoy it. BANFEBA Meditation is a technique to keep you on this track, transcending thought, always pulling you back into the peaceful feeling of Being. Once we are totally awake to Being, which has always been there, the peaceful feeling of Being will always be there.

The High of Enlightenment

There are other artificial ways to induce a more accepting, transcendental mode of awareness, but they all have adverse consequences. Drinking alcohol is the most popular. 70% of people in America drink alcohol at least three times a week. Recreational drug use is less socially accepted, but it is still a major presence in the world today.

There is currently a lot of research in the media proving drinking a glass or two of wine each day is good for your heart, and drinking alcohol in moderation allows you to live longer. If you research people presently living the longest in the world, in the "Blue Zones,"[8] you will discover a lot of them drink wine. Besides releasing stress, wine also has many anti-oxidants in it, which fight disease. The combination of those benefits, according to the research, helps us live longer. However, the alcohol in wine is, chemically, a poison that destroys brain cells, pollutes your liver, and strains your nervous system. A hangover from drinking alcohol (in any form) is the tangible evidence of what is physically and mentally harmful about drinking alcohol. Your experience will quickly teach you that alcohol is definitely not a panacea to perfect health.

Step Four: FEEL

The quandary we face in life is we are all a lot more addicted to feeling high, than we may admit. We are all innately programmed to release stress to feel higher. Addiction, at whatever level, is an addiction to feeling higher. Life is not about just making it through in one piece. Life is about living fully and totally enjoying it. Our natural tendency toward trying to be happy no matter how we get there is an indication of our natural tendency to evolve to higher states of consciousness. The problem is we are using the wrong methods of feeling higher because, although consuming wine may have some health benefits, on balance alcohol consumption has too many negative side effects.

Alcohol addiction, even moderate addiction, comes with an undeniable cost. The World Health Organization says that every year 2.5 million people die from alcohol abuse, but there is no revolution against drinking. Why? Because getting high, drinking, feels really good, and we all love to feel good.

What are we to do? Well, don't give up your beer or your glass of wine; just add meditation. Once you start becoming higher naturally, you will feel less need to supplement the high, artificially, and it is a much clearer high. The more you meditate, the more you will become aware that alcohol and drugs numb your senses. Meditation does just the opposite. You become more sensitive to the beauty of life. You feel high on life, and your senses are picking up all the details you have previously missed.

Once you become more aware of your body, you will feel exactly what the alcohol is doing to you. Alcohol in alcoholic drinks is a toxic chemical called ethanol. Ethanol is a poison. It is a chemical depressant. You are killing brain cells after the initial high, and you spend most of the time coming down off the high in a depressed state. Drugs can be even more destructive to your nervous system depending on the particular drug, and the level of use. The brilliant actor, Philip Seymour Hoffman, died using heroin. He was only 46. He is famous, so we all heard about it, but there are so many more people, dying each day from drug use, we don't hear about. Turn on the news; presently, there is a horrendous epidemic of pharmaceutical opioid abuse in America.

I say all of this without preaching from the stump. I, too, as a teenager, experimented with alcohol and drugs. Some people have to go further down the alcohol – drug path than others to learn, but eventually, over time, life will direct you to the same path we are all, ultimately, on – the path to enlightenment. The good news is – enlightenment feels extremely good, and once you head down that path, and have the actual experience, you will find it is much easier to abandon alcohol and drugs because you won't miss them at all. The high of enlightenment is completely holistic and healthy.

The Paradox of Sex

The paradox of sex is, while making love can be a blissful expression of God allowing a new soul to enter this world, the experience of sexual intercourse can also easily become addicting, distorted, and decadent slowing us down from experiencing enlightenment.

There is a lot of contradiction surrounding sex on our spiritual paths. Sex is always a tricky subject in spiritual books because it stirs up so much controversy. Many priests, holy men, gurus, and spiritual teachers from all different religions and faiths have been shamed and ruined by their association with sex.

I, personally, am unrepentantly waving my flag high to say, yes, I have lived a life complete with numerous sexual relationships. I believe it was an integral part of becoming who I am now. It was fun. I enjoyed it, and it didn't ruin me.

Step Four: FEEL

Siddhartha Gautama had many sexual relationships before he eventually reached enlightenment so I believed I ultimately could too. Sexual experience is not a prerequisite on the path to enlightenment, but it won't stop you either. I am now happily married to my beautiful wife, Sheila, and we have an amazing son, Weston.

We are each unique people on different paths, and each of those paths is valid. Follow your experience. Experience is your teacher. Always be awake to what your experience is teaching you. If you are feeling blissful and happy during and after sex, and you are able to maintain that delicate balance, then continue. However, if you are feeling drained of energy, and filled with negative emotions then take a different path, and refrain from sex. An exclusively platonic relationship may be completely fulfilling for you if the mutual love is strong enough.

Sex can be a beautiful expression of being totally alive. Repression of sexual desires may, if not channeled properly, lead to emotional problems that may eventually express themselves in unhealthy ways. The controversy surrounding numerous celibate Catholic priests exemplifies one of the many possible negative effects of sexual repression over an extended period. However, let's also remember the majority of priests have devoted their lives to working in the service of God, and their path of celibacy may have worked well for them just as it may have worked well for many celibate Hindu and Buddhist monks.

Like drugs and alcohol, one must always keep an eye on sex, because the high of sex can also become addicting and destructive. Our egos feed off of sexual addiction, and that may slow you down from reaching your goal of enlightenment. Our egos will focus our energy in one location – our lower selves. Instead, we need to experience Being, which is our Higher Self, always flowing, never contained, and universal.

According to ancient Indian knowledge from the Vedas, in our bodies, we have seven main energy centers, called chakras, lined up from the base of our spine to the top of our head. When energy collects in those different chakras, we have a different experience or feeling. Our second chakra, or Sacral Chakra, is located in the pelvic area, and when energy collects there, we feel sexually excited. When, through our spiritual practice, we become more connected to the infinite source of energy, that new energy has to express itself somewhere, and many times you will find it appearing as sexual urges.

As you reach higher states of consciousness, your sexual desires may increase until finally you are awake enough to transcend your desires. The key is not to always direct the extra energy to your second chakra, or it will become a habit. It is like going to the bank, getting lots of cash, but always just buying chocolate. Chocolate is great, but there are many other great things in life to spend our money on.

Making love to someone you cherish is a beautiful, profound, spiritual experience. However, ego-induced sex, which is much more common, can easily lead you in the opposite direction, and it's a trap that is so easy to fall victim to. Our culture is immersed in sexual decadence. Music, movies, TV, books, and the Internet all constantly feed off our innate desire for sex. Ultimately, as long as you are not harming anyone, it makes no difference what specifically arouses you sexually, but sex can slow down your evolution toward enlightenment if you allow it to become addicting.

If you study Ayurveda, knowledge from the Vedas, home of Yoga and ancient Vedic meditation techniques, you will discover the seed of our Being, the essence of who we are on this physical plane is distilled in our bodies as a substance called Ojas. Ojas collects in the heart. Ojas is also the life force at the core of semen. The more we ejaculate, the more we deplete our Ojas.

Step Four: FEEL

The more enlightened we are, the more Ojas we have. If you want to reach enlightenment faster, learn to retain your semen more, and stay in balance.

If you study ancient Tantra sexual techniques, you will find ways to enjoy sex, and experience orgasm, without ejaculating. Those techniques work, however, that practice can also become addicting. The practice increases sexual thoughts, which are the seeds of sexual experience, and the cycle of increasing attachment to your ego is reinforced.

In the real world, how do we deal with this sexual conundrum? The best path is to use meditation to balance your sexual activity. BANFEBA is the key to allowing you to transcend all desires including an overpowering sex drive. *As soon as a sexual thought appears, accept it, transcend it, feel, and experience Being instead. The key is to not allow the chain of sexual thoughts to continue, or you will find yourself attached to those thoughts, and you will eventually act on it. Stop the process at the beginning.* When you transcend sexual desires, which lead to sexual activity – it will stop the desire for sex before it becomes too strong to control. The good news is the high you then feel, as your energy builds every day, is like a never-ending subtle, blissful orgasm, so you don't have an overpowering sexual drive. Instead, you will have a continual feeling of bliss and happiness. *By using the Seven Steps, you will eventually be able to transcend all desires because you will feel so amazing you will not have the desire to experience anything else but Being.*

The more you practice this process, and balance your sexual drive, the easier it gets. However, when the special moment does come when you decide to join your life force with another human in a bond of love, enjoy the experience of sex to the fullest. *The euphoric experience of sexual orgasm is a profound taste of enlightenment. It is the seed used to create another human being. That is the evidence of its enormous divine power.*

Rich, Famous, and Powerful

Struggling in life to become rich, famous, and powerful has always been portrayed in spiritual books as the antithesis of searching for enlightenment. However, it is important not for us to be self-righteous, and judge others. Remember, ultimately, at our core, we are all the same.

The reason so many people on earth continually seek substantial wealth, fame and power is because the feeling superficially mimics the experience of enlightenment. Most of us had a time in our lives when we got paid for a big job, and we are flush with cash. The sudden influx of money allows a brief feeling of contentment. The stress of paying our bills temporarily vanishes. We now have the ability to realize our dreams. We go out to a special restaurant to celebrate. We go on a vacation. We buy that amazing new car, or maybe we even buy that perfect house we always dreamed of. When we are rich many of our desires are instantly fulfilled.

Have you recently noticed that everybody now also wants, not only to be rich but to be famous too? We seek out as many friends as we can on Facebook, Instagram, Twitter, and all of the other social media platforms. We post pictures of ourselves, displaying our exciting lives, searching for acclaim from our new "friends." Is this phenomena really new? No, everybody has always wanted to feel infinitely connected to all people. We just never had the technology, or the ability, to do it before. We have always wanted to feel totally connected to all other people because it is a taste of enlightenment.

Have you ever noticed that everyone struggles to climb the career ladder to be the boss, but on the way up, we all complain about the boss? Employees are always yearning to be the boss because it makes us powerful, and being powerful allows us freedom, and the ability to satisfy our desires. When we are powerful, our superficial desires are created faster. We want

Step Four: FEEL

something, we ask someone to go get it for us, and it arrives immediately. Being the boss gives us power, but it is limited, and it is superficial. Enlightenment connects us with infinite, unlimited, real power. We become the boss of our entire life. We all have an innate desire for infinite power because, ultimately, we are at our core, infinitely powerful. Power, like money, is neither good nor bad, it is only how we use power or money that makes it good or bad.

The initial feeling of being rich, famous, and powerful is great, but it usually doesn't last long, and it always comes with baggage. We want more, so we fight to get it again. When we do get it, it never completely satisfies us. Being rich, famous, or powerful is a transient experience we will never be able to maintain, and it is never as great as we imagine it to be. There is always something missing in the experience. Even presidents, rock stars, movie stars, and sports stars are eventually put out to pasture. Their fame becomes obscure, their fortunes diminish, and the items they continue to buy don't fulfill them anymore.

There is always something missing in the experience of life until we are fully enlightened. When we are enlightened, we have a complete feeling of contentment, happiness, unity, and power, and the feeling is eternal. Our important desires are created effortlessly. We get what we need in life. We are connected to all other people on the planet; the experience feels absolute and powerful. That is what we really desire. There are no bad side effects with enlightenment. Perpetually fighting, and struggling to be rich, famous, or powerful has so many obvious pitfalls. Enlightenment, however, will fulfill us in ways that money, fame, and power never can. This is not some sanctimonious proclamation; it is a tangible fact. Stay awake, and allow your experience to teach you it is true.

Funny

We all love to laugh, and we love to make others laugh. Laughing is a pure byproduct of Being. Laughing feels great. Tests have proven that people that laugh profusely live longer, healthier, happier lives. We flock to movies that make us laugh. We search TV, and the Internet for funny skits, and situations. Talented comedians are special stars that we all love.

In my house, comedy is king. My son, Weston, my wife, Sheila, and I are constantly cracking jokes, and acting like clowns to get each other to laugh. That is a good thing because it makes our lives fun, and happy. But even jokes, like movies, skits on TV, and the Internet deliver laughs that are temporary. They don't last. We all want to laugh and feel happy continually. Enlightenment will allow you to experience happiness without any outside stimulus. You will spontaneously laugh a lot, and it feels fantastic. You will spontaneously find humor in everyday life.

The Science of Euphoria

I'm not a scientist, but I have been experimenting my whole life. I have experimented with drugs, alcohol, success, money, power, extreme sports, and sex. I have observed they all have one thing in common; initially, they feel great. They are also totally addicting, and when they are out of balance, they can completely ruin your life.

Drugs, alcohol, success, money, power, extreme sports, and sex increase neurotransmitters and hormones in our brains. They increase dopamine, serotonin, oxytocin, and endorphins; the chemicals in your brain, that are responsible for your happiness. The increase of these chemicals makes us feel amazing. The process is more complex than this simple explanation, but basically, the euphoric feeling serotonin, dopamine, and other neurotransmitters create is what we are all fighting for in almost everything we do, whether we know it or not. The problem with drugs, alcohol, success, money, power, extreme sports and sex is the euphoric feeling is temporary, and if they are not kept in proper balance, each of those pathways will eventually lead to destruction.

The good news is you can get that same great feeling from neurotransmitters and hormones without any negative side effects. Science has proven that serotonin, dopamine, oxytocin, and endorphins levels are increased dramatically during meditation, and meditation is holistic, in perfect balance, and life supporting. Research the relationship between meditation, neurotransmitters, and hormones, and you will find this analysis is correct. There is an abundance of science that validates the many benefits of meditation. Meditation increases serotonin, dopamine, oxytocin, endorphins, and DHEA. The result is we are much happier, healthier, and we will live longer, but my advice is for you to experiment with meditation yourself. Experience meditation and you will actually feel the incredible results.

Food for Enlightenment

Feeling Being is essential to moving forward on the path to enlightenment. The actual feeling of Being is extremely subtle at first, and if you are not sensitive to your physical body, you will completely miss it. Without the right nutrition, you will stay numb to those finer feelings.

If you are going to commit to reaching enlightenment, you must start eating healthy. Specifically, that means you should try your best to eat organic, natural foods that have not been processed in any way. The food industry has learned how to increase profits well by feeding our innate addiction to sugar, salt, and fat. Look around you, and you will see the evidence is everywhere. Look at the ingredients before you eat anything.

Sugar, in various forms, is the biggest culprit, and it is literally in every form of processed food. Sugar is as addicting as cocaine, so we always want more. Sugar negatively affects your moods, your metabolism, and your immune system.

What you eat, directly affects your body, your health, and your happiness. Carnivores may not want to hear this, but if you want to reach enlightenment fast, you should become a vegan. Dead meat vibrates at a very low frequency. It also embodies a lot of negative consciousness because of the way the animals are slaughtered. On top of that, meat is killing you, too, slowly.

There have been numerous studies including a recent study by the World Health Organization where 18 scientists from 17 different countries all concluded processed meat leads directly to cancer, and all meat "probably" does too. If you want further proof of how eating meat is harming you, read – *The China Study*. The New York Times called it the most comprehensive nutrition study ever conducted.

The China Study proves eating animal protein leads directly to the number one killer in America – heart disease, and the number two killer – cancer; plus stroke, diabetes, and so many other diseases it is hard to list here. If you are a hardcore carnivore, as I was before the age of 16, then ride both trains for a while. Start practicing BANFEBA Meditation, and continue to enjoy your steak, but keep an eye open to how you really feel. Your experience will eventually teach you. Follow your experience.

What you eat is extremely important on your path to enlightenment, but so is how much you eat. Obesity is currently rampant in America due to our bad food choices, but also due to our large food portions. If you study Ayurveda, knowledge from the Vedas, you will discover that you should only fill your stomach up three-quarters of the way, leaving enough room for proper digestion. Think of the food as logs in a fire. If we put too many logs in the fire, we will snuff it out. We need to allow more oxygen to increase the strength of the fire. Japanese culture promotes the same smaller food portion theory; they call it, "hara hachi bun me," a Confucian teaching that instructs people to only eat until they are 80 percent full. It is no accident that Japanese people are generally skinnier, and they have a longer lifespan than people in America. Japanese people eat more vegetables and much smaller portions than we do in America. Your body is your instrument to experience higher levels of consciousness, so you need to constantly refine it, and keep it in optimal health.

The Feeling of Enlightenment is Eternal

The biggest irony of moving forward on the path to enlightenment is that the analytical mind, logically, is trying to understand the process of how to reach enlightenment. Your mind will evolve extensively as you become more awake, but it will never be able to completely comprehend an enlightened state of consciousness.

It is physically impossible for our limited minds to totally understand an infinite source of knowledge. However, we can experience it, we can feel it, and that will be enough to fulfill you. In fact, once you are experiencing Being on a regular basis, you will then have no desire to totally understand it; instead it will be like you are living in a marvelous movie you love so much, you never want it to end. The good news is – it won't end. *Once you become totally awake to your identification with Being, the experience of enlightenment will be eternal.*

Your Body is Your Vehicle to Feel Enlightenment

Keeping your body healthy is essential to maintaining higher states of consciousness. Eating lots of organic, fresh fruits and vegetables, daily exercise, drinking lots of water, and getting enough sleep, all dramatically affect the moods, and the consciousness we are experiencing. When your body is healthy, you will experience higher states of consciousness much easier. Take it one step at a time. The Seven Steps will work no matter what else you do, but you can either run uphill to get to your destination, or you can run downhill, or you can strap wings to your back and fly. It all depends on how fast you want to get there.

Aging is a Feeling

In 2008, I filmed and directed a documentary, *Aging in America*. We never completed the film, but through the process, I learned a lot. I traveled across America from New York to Los Angeles, for three months, interviewing doctors, scientists, and legions of elderly people to research the story behind *Aging in America*.

I even had the opportunity during the 2008, presidential election in Iowa, to briefly meet and film President Barack Obama, Secretary of State Hillary Clinton, former President Bill Clinton, Senator John McCain, and Governor Mitt Romney. As well-intentioned, and engaging as each of these political leaders were, none of them had a comprehensive agenda or strategy for taking care of the elderly in America, which is quickly becoming our countries largest demographic.

Poor health in America is a paramount problem, and we need to seriously engage holistic solutions as a matter of national policy as our country continues to age. What is a holistic solution for taking care of the elderly? We need to age slower and more naturally, by changing our daily habits to become healthier. We need to restore natural balance to our bodies. We need to eat well, exercise and meditate. We need to meditate to release stress and create a positive mindset. Modern medicine has already validated the incredible health benefits of meditation. We need to allow the natural flow of the Universe to keep us in balance and healthy. Without the natural support of Being, most people spend much of their lives slowly decaying and slowly dying. Feel Being, and you will feel younger and more vibrant, and your body will naturally reflect that. There is so much scientific research that validates the many benefits of meditation, and yet, we always just relegate it to a negligible position in our health care system. We need to change that. We need to make meditation a priority.

Feel the Glow of Being

When you feel absolute peace within, without thinking about it or labeling it, you are feeling Being, the Source of all creation. Continue doing this as much as possible, until it becomes a habit. Feeling is an entry point to the connection with the Source. If you can't feel Being, take a deep breath. Still can't transcend your thinking mind? Accept the thinking.

Accept whatever you are presently feeling, even if your mind has labeled it "bad" – accept it anyway, and feel it. Feel it until you feel Being subtly, behind the thinking, at the core. Feel Being until it transforms your state of consciousness. Be aware of the peaceful feeling of Being, and you will feel contentment and love.

Maharishi used to describe the feeling of Being as, "The Glow." I love that expression. Being does glow, and when you are connected to Being, you glow with an effervescent sparkle in your eyes, and the actual feeling is one of glowing with peace and love. Eternal, infinite, peace, and fulfillment are the feeling of Being – you and the Universe glowing as one. *Breathe and Accept the Now; Feel and Experience Being Awareness*

Chapter Five

Step Five
EXPERIENCE

BANFEBA Meditation is a natural process that allows you to transcend thinking to experience Being Awareness. The experience of Being is more than just feeling it. The experience expands to encompass all five senses. As we begin to experience more of Being, the experience is even more than can be felt, heard, tasted, smelled, and seen. It becomes a transcendental experience. Feeling Being is the beginning, but the experience of Being is infinite. The experience is so profound it is impossible to describe completely with words.

In order to experience Being follow the first four steps, then allow the experience of Being to be natural and effortless. Breathe, accept the now, feel, and experience Being. You experience Being by allowing Being to be experienced. Don't try to find it, allow it to come to you. Don't chase it, or try to manipulate it. Become awake to the fact that it is already there. The deep peace of Being is the core experience, but Being is

Step Five: EXPERIENCE

experienced in our relative lives in infinite ways, all of them profound.

As you start to experience that you are more than what your ego has created, and you identify more with Being, your world will completely change in a positive direction. You will experience more peace, contentment, and happiness. You will experience the world as a reflection of Being. *At its source, Being is experienced as pure silence and peace. In the relative world, we live in; Being is experienced as love, happiness, and bliss.* The experience of Being can most easily be felt internally, but Being is Universal. It is always there, everywhere. *Being is always within you, and surrounding you. Being is omnipresent.*

Effortlessly shift your attention to your awareness, until you can actually experience Being. As the process progresses, you will become more aware of the experience. It will start off being very subtle. Eventually, you will become more awake to your expanded sense of self. The boundary limiting your inner self will dissolve. *You will eventually recognize and experience you are everything you see, touch, and feel.* You will actually experience yourself as part of the Universe, and you will realize that has always been, and it always will be your true identity.

The Vedic Sanskrit mantra, Aham Brahmasmi, translated means, "I am the Universe." You are the Universe because the Source of you is Being, and Being is the Source of the Universe. Those may feel like awfully big shoes to fill, but we can literally experience as much of that truth as we allow ourselves. Once you have the experience of a profound awareness of Being, your true identity will become more evident.

When you walk on the beach, through the woods, or climb a mountain, the experience of oneness with the Universe is easier to comprehend, but you can experience Being, and a sense of oneness, literally anywhere. Ultimately, that taste of enlightenment is not something you need to comprehend fully, it is only something you need to experience. Direct your attention to Being. Feel Being. Experience Being. Feel it without thinking about what you are feeling. If you feel tired, despondent, anxious, or complacent, just feel whatever is there now. As you put your attention on the feeling of Being, you will become aware that the feeling will naturally transform until it is peaceful. Put your attention on the peace that surrounds you and realize it is an extension of your own Being. There are no boundaries of Being. Being is eternal and infinite. Experience it. Identify with that experience. Being is who you really are. You are a part of Being. Don't identify with the experience of your lower-self created by your ego that bounces like a life raft on the ocean up and down – happy, not happy; sad, not sad; angry, not angry. *Experience and identify with Being.* Being is like the lighthouse, securely built on a solid rock overlooking the ocean, with its bright light witnessing the ocean oscillating, bobbing up and down, but always feeling secure with its solid foundation.

Identify With Your Higher Self Through Experience

Most people here on Earth only recognize and therefore experience their lower self, the thinking mind, the ego, experiencing the relative world they have created for themselves. BANFEBA Meditation is a technique to allow your Higher Self to experience Being. *Your true identity is your individual awareness, your Higher Self, experiencing infinite, eternal Being.*

Identification With Our Ego Will Lead Us to Destruction

The identity our ego has created for us in this lifetime will always end up being destroyed eventually by death, and smaller stages of destruction will happen periodically throughout our life.

We may have an accident. A crash may destroy our car. A fire may burn down our kitchen, or our whole house. We may catch a disease and spend a portion of our lives fighting it. We may become addicted to alcohol, or drugs, and destroy our health. Our girlfriend or boyfriend may leave us and break our heart. Our wife or husband may leave us and ruin our marriage. Our parents might get divorced and put immense stress on our childhood. We could fail in school, or at our new job. Our business might fail. We may go bankrupt. We may get into an altercation that gets physical, and we may end up in jail.

Fortunately, most of us don't experience all of the situations mentioned above, but I am sure all of us have experienced one or two, or maybe several of those situations. Destruction is a natural part of life. We are born, we live for a while, and then we die. Everything in life follows the same natural pattern. The plants, the animals, even the planet we live on, will eventually be destroyed. Destruction is part of the natural cycle of life. Being, however, is absolute. *Being is invincible. Being is eternal.*

Being is Invincible

Sometimes destruction can become overwhelming because we identify only with the limited part of ourselves, that our egos have created. We identify with our names, our bodies, our situations in life. However, that part of our identity is only temporary, and because we falsely identify with that part of ourselves, we feel pain when it is destroyed.

We will continue to experience the pain of our lives being destroyed until we recognize and experience the peace of Being as the Source of who we really are. *Our true identities are perfect eternal Beings presently living temporary experiences in temporary bodies.* We are perfect eternal Beings, but we will only experience that perfection when we experience Being. Nothing can destroy Being. When we become awake to, and experience, our identity as part of Being, we naturally feel secure and invincible.

Once we experience Being instead of just our egos, our lives will reflect that, and we will become healthier, happier, and more content. That feeling of security gives us a lot of confidence in life. Our lives may still follow the relative life cycle of ups and downs, but we will not be totally affected by it. We will witness the changes from a perspective of truth, peace, and even happiness. Yes, you can even experience peace when destruction is simultaneously experienced in your life. This is not just a positive mindset. It is a tangible reality. *Being is invincible, experience it, identify with it, and you will also become invincible.*

Return to Being

Being is our home. Always return home. We must always direct our awareness back to Being. It is so easy to get hijacked by our desires, or a situation, or someone else's energy. It is so easy to get caught up in the drama of the moment. The collective consciousness of humanity is a field of energy we are always immersed in and affected by.

If we walk into a bar or a football stadium, we feel one way; if we walk into a church, a temple, or a library, we feel another. It is true of any space we enter filled with people. People's thoughts collect like invisible clouds, interacting, linking up, and those thoughts affect the way we think.

Don't fight the thoughts, always remember, we are not our thoughts. We are an expression of Being, witnessing our thoughts. *Our thoughts are like a river that flows past. Don't identify with the thoughts, and don't try to stop them. Instead, we must accept our thoughts to transcend our thoughts and return home to the feeling and experience of Being.*

Take a deep breath; accept whatever is happening right now, feel and experience Being. *Feel and experience whatever is happening to you right now. Accept it. Don't judge it or fight*

Step Five: EXPERIENCE

it. Accept it, feel it, and experience it within you. *The experience will transform into the pure peace of Being.* Identify with that experience of peace. It is the real you.

Inner Feeling Reflects Outer Life

What we are currently feeling actually creates what we are experiencing in the world. If we are feeling good, the world appears happy and beautiful. If we are angry and upset, the world is experienced as mean, cold, and ugly. Try it out. Keep your attention on your feelings, and then take note of how the world appears to you. Your experience will teach you.

Once you realize this is true, you will know you are the master of your own world. BANFEBA Meditation is a key to creating a better world. The Seven Steps will allow you to return to a better feeling and experience. Experience Being and your world will become beautiful, happy, and fulfilling.

The Path to Heaven

Don't ever be scared of death. Being is eternal. Your experience of Being is eternal. Identify with Being. You are part of Being. Your life is eternal. When you die, you leave your body, but you can still see, and experience life – you move to a higher realm of life, Heaven, where everything is incredibly beautiful, and it feels absolutely amazing.

Our fear of death holds us back in our life on Earth. Our fear keeps us from experiencing life to its fullest. Once your awareness awakens through BANFEBA Meditation, you will start to partially experience, and understand life in these higher realms. That deep awareness will also allow you to live life here more fully because you won't be scared of dying. The ego is scared of death because everything your ego has created is temporary, and death is the end of it all. Identify with Being, and then you will not be scared of death because Being is eternal.

Those who die will be in Heaven, and if we are awake enough, we can still communicate with them. Telepathic communication is rarely like a voice on the phone, it is mostly an absolute feeling where you totally understand every word, but you didn't hear anything audible. However, it all depends on how clear your awareness is. When you are totally aware of Being the experience will be very clear. You will know exactly what they are saying. Spirits usually only want one thing – to express their deep love for their family, and the friends they have left behind. They always want them to know they are okay, and it is beautiful where they are. They want their families and friends to live happy lives, not to cry for them, and for them to know – they will always love them.

In my life, I have experienced that loss several times. I have witnessed both of my parents die, and I have known several friends who died early in their life. I am sure many of you have experienced that loss also. It is sad because sometimes we feel like they and their family were cheated, but we must always remember life is eternal. They were not cheated. They just needed to move on in order to evolve faster on a different plane of existence. *The game of life is completely set up for us to reach enlightenment. Our unique lives are individually set up for us to become awake to whom we really are. Being constantly guides us toward that reality.* From our limited point of view, we will ask: why did he or she die? How can there be a God if a great young man or woman was taken from his or her family so early? It never seems fair. We see reprehensible people live into old age and some of our very best are taken so early. Well, the answer to that particular equation is some graduate from school early, and some need to stay in school longer.

Life is precious, and we should value every heartbeat and every breath. However, when you die you go to a place so fantastic, and so full of love and beauty, you will be absolutely thrilled you have arrived. You will eventually come back to Earth with an evolved perspective. The cycle continues until you are fully enlightened. Once you are enlightened, your life will still continue, but there is no interruption of your awareness. You become awake to your eternal life.

Heaven is not up in the clouds; Heaven is within you, and surrounding you. It is on another frequency of existence most people can't see. When we die, and our ego is not interfering, we are able to experience Heaven. Heaven is real. Heaven is absolute pure Being. *To become aware of Being, here now, is your path to living Heaven on Earth.*

Being is a Tangible Experience

Being is not a philosophical concept or a manufactured ideology, it is a tangible experience. Being is absolute silence and deep peace. Being is pure awareness, without thoughts. It is a feeling that transcends your experience of you, but you can feel it, personally, glowing in your body. It is the feeling of complete fulfillment.

There is no ego attached and no feeling of ownership. It is only positive, blissful, and loving. You have to experience Being to understand it, and even then you will only understand it on an intuitive level. Being is infinite, but the actual experience of Being will feel complete and totally fulfilling.

Experience Being to Transcend the Battles of Life

Most of the time in our normal, day-to-day lives we don't feel this deep experience of Being, we only experience the problems facing us. Misidentification is the cause of all feelings of doubt, fear, jealousy, greed, lust, anger, and anxiety. Our thinking minds, controlled by our egos, have blinded us to our true Selves. We continually identify only with our egos, and we fight to defend our lower selves created by our egos.

We habitually think another person is attacking us or treating us wrong, and we need to defend ourselves, or they will continue. We look at life as a battle, fighting for respect, love, and money or any other desire we have concocted that we think is imperative. We break up into different groups of people, joining people in one camp who have similar thinking patterns, and we fight people in other camps where they think differently. Those camps can be countries, states, companies, religions, gangs, etc. Even sports teams can fall victim to the war camp mentality.

The problem is no one camp will ever win, or if it does, it will eventually meet failure, because individuals in the camp will not fundamentally be experiencing the reality of life. We, human beings, fail to recognize, ultimately, we are all connected and part of a whole. We are all coming from and going to the same place. We are one. Our souls are connected. The core of who we each are is the same.

Of course, you may understand this concept theoretically, but when someone cuts you off on the highway, or almost runs you over in a crosswalk, or insults you, you immediately feel angry. That is okay. Just use the anger as an indicator you are identifying with the ego.

Take a deep breath, accept the anger, feel it, and allow the feeling to transform into the experience of Being. Become aware of the peaceful feeling of Being, experience it, and then you will automatically, effortlessly, smile. You have changed your identification, and that has allowed you to transcend the thinking, angry mind. Feel Being, which is always peaceful and experience Being; that is who you really are.

Acceptance Leads to the Experience of Being

The key is not to think, oh I am not where I want to be, and I am not feeling the way I want to feel. I felt so perfect when I was walking on the beach this morning or when I was doing yoga,

Step Five: EXPERIENCE

or playing with my children, or some other special activity, but now I am not. The key is to transcend your desires, and accept the Now, to experience Being.

Accept exactly how you are thinking and feeling right now. Accept you are angry, accept you are frustrated, accept you are feeling sick, accept you are lonely, bored, unfulfilled, unhappy, judgmental, or conversely, accept you are feeling proud, happy, honored, satisfied. Accept what you are feeling right now, and that will allow you to transcend thinking, feel, and experience Being. *The more you experience Being, the more you will continue to experience Being.*

Experience God

Beyond matter, all things known and unknown in our relative world, there is an absolute, peaceful, dynamic field of energy that is the Source of all creation. It is infinite and so vast and comprehensive it is beyond words or descriptions. It can be felt and experienced through BANFEBA meditation, but it is unfathomable to the human mind. The key is not to try to totally understand it, because no one ever completely will, but to recognize we are expressions of it, we are part of it, and to experience it as much as possible. It is Being. It is God.

In the *International Version of the Bible*, it says, "I pray that out of his glorious riches he may strengthen you with power through his Spirit in your inner Being."[9] That clearly means if you become awake to your inner Being you will experience God. Put it to the test – feel Being, and you will experience God.

Enlightenment is a state of profound awareness, where one experiences Being. Being is already at the core of your natural state of awareness. However, the mind, which is controlled by the ego, has clouded most people's awareness, so they only experience the feeling of Being in rare glimpses, and even then they are not aware of what they are truly feeling. An enlightened level of awareness is totally tangible. You can actually feel it as a subtle, but profound, dynamic energy within your body and surrounding you. You will notice it in the way you see and perceive things, the way you hear different sounds, music, voices, and nature. Everything is more pronounced, crystal clear, and you can feel and understand the subtle interconnection of everything in the Universe. You can feel the deep silence and peace within all things.

The more that deep core of peace is experienced in our relative world the more we will feel a profound feeling of deep peace, love, and bliss, and we will recognize that is our true identity.

Life is Relative; Being is Absolute

When you become more awake, and you start experiencing enlightenment, it doesn't mean your life is not going to face any more troubles. We all live in a relative state of existence. There will always be ups and downs in life. The difference is when you are living in an enlightened state, you will have the ability to transcend the unwanted feelings and emotions. You will witness the challenging experiences, but you are always, simultaneously, able to experience a deep peace within.

You still got the parking ticket for neglecting to feed the meter because you were having too good of time having chai tea with a new friend, but you accept the fine. The fine rolls off you like a bead of water off a duck. You know you're okay, and you feel okay, so you don't worry. Even if your trouble is bigger than a parking ticket, you still can handle it. Live in the present moment, and you will soon recognize almost all of your troubles are in your perceived future. You have enough money now to pay the ticket, you are only worried about running out of money in your future.

Just transcend any desires, accept the Now, and enjoy it. When you live this way, consciously breathing when you run into a snag, or when you just want to feel better, you will start to notice your life is changing for the better in the relative level of existence. You will notice good things start happening to you. You experience "good luck" often. Things start going your way. Your bad day can end up being as good as your old good days used to be, and your new good days will be fantastic. Life will still be relative, but never awful.

Experience a Vision of God

Can we actually reach such a profound state of awareness we can experience God? Yes, we can actually catch a glimpse of the infinite Source if we are awake enough.

When I was seventeen years old, I was invited on a winter mountaineering expedition to climb the highest mountain in Wyoming, Gannett Peak. At an elevation of 13,809 ft., Gannett is considered one of the hardest mountains to climb in the United States. I had already climbed Gannett and five other of the highest mountains in the Wind River Range in Wyoming the summer before, but this time, we wanted to reach the summit on New Year's day. No one had ever climbed Gannett in the winter before, and there is a good reason for that. Gannett is extremely cold in the winter, in a very remote part of one of the largest wilderness areas in the United States. There is an abundance of snow and ice.

As we started our climb, the temperature was forty below zero, Fahrenheit. It was so cold our spit would literally freeze before it hit the ground. We hiked into the deep snow on mountain skis, toward Gannett, deep into the wilderness for five days, camping at night in such cold weather you were thankful to even see the sun in the morning. It was incredibly cold, but also stunningly beautiful.

Then a blizzard hit us. We couldn't move further into the wilderness, and after being stuck for two days, we only had enough supplies left for one more day of climbing. We had to reset our target to Fremont Peak, Wyoming's third highest Mountain, which was within climbing distance the next day if the weather cleared.

We woke up to a beautiful sunny morning and started climbing. Of our five climbers, one had terrible blisters that were now bleeding, one had a broken ski, and our guide, Courtney Skinner, who was a legendary mountaineer as a young man, declared, three quarters of the way to the summit, he was too exhausted from the altitude to make the final dash to the top.

One other climber, Chris and I saw by the low angle of the sun in the sky, we had about two hours left to reach the summit, and get off the mountain before the darkness made it impossible to navigate. So we climbed as fast as possible. We were at 13,000 feet, and my thinking was clouded. At high altitudes, you actually start feeling almost intoxicated and sometimes act irrationally. I was only seventeen years old, but I was racing up the mountain as fast as I could in order to gain the glory of being the first to climb Fremont in the winter.

I figured we were about thirty feet from the top, but the actual summit of Fremont peak was hard to distinguish because it is so broad, especially in the winter when it was covered in snow, and at sunset with low light. It was hard to tell if part of the ridge was higher or lower. I had already reached the summit the summer before, but now it all felt completely different. Chris, who was a few years older, and a more experienced climber, declared this was close enough to the top to claim victory, and we should now get the hell off this mountain before the sun completely set, and we died up there.

I told Chris I wanted to continue to climb, and he responded, that it was pointless and not necessary; we had made it to the top. He was probably right, but my ego wanted to be absolutely certain. He dismissed my argument, and he started climbing

Step Five: EXPERIENCE

down ahead of me. I didn't move. I looked at the ridge, still trying to determine if we were high enough to claim victory. I was frustrated because my ego wanted to make certain I was victorious. I then, reluctantly, continued down after him. I was angry, and I was climbing recklessly. It was getting darker, and I fell. It was only a short fall of about ten feet, but it was enough to snap me back to reality; I could easily die up here.

I stopped. I took a deep breath. I let it all go, and I accepted everything completely. I looked out to see the sun setting over the mountains. I then saw one of the most spectacular sights I have ever seen. Hanging in the orange glowing sky above the sun, was an expansive glowing cloud type formation that looked exactly like a beautiful angel with piercing eyes. It was completely translucent, with a bright light shining through, and the experience of being in its presence was breathtaking. I stared at it, mesmerized by its beauty until finally, I realized I had better continue climbing. It was such an amazing experience. Instantly, I could care less whether I had reached the actual summit or not. The experience was so profound. I felt totally fulfilled.

A cynic could easily dismiss the event as a cloud my imagination, amplified by the altitude, had contrived into an angel formation. However, several years later, I found an old book in a small bookstore in Iowa, *The Kingdom of the Gods*, by Geoffrey Hodson, first published in 1952 in India. In that book, I found an exact picture of my angel. Hobson calls it a Mountain God. He used the Kabbalistic term, "Sephira." He describes the beings as expressions of God that inhabit Nature on our planet. They can occasionally be seen by the human eye if we are awake enough.

That was a transformational moment in my life. Chris and I reconnected with Courtney, halfway down the face of the mountain. The sun was down, the temperature was dropping fast, and we were completely exhausted. I knew I couldn't make it all the way back to the base camp, but for some reason, I wasn't scared. Courtney could tell we were physically spent, and he led us to the bank of a frozen mountain lake, where he started probing in the deep snow with his ice ax.

Miraculously, he found an opening, and we climbed in to find an ice cave, built early that winter by a group of explorers from National Geographic. Courtney had visited the explorers earlier in the winter, and incredibly, he remembered where the caves were. When we entered the ice cave, it was like slipping into a warm house. The cave was the temperature of the snow, around 28 degrees, and compared with forty below zero outside it felt like a sauna. I am convinced the ice cave saved my life, and I am also convinced the Mountain God helped us find it.

Other mountain climbers, long distance sailors, astronauts, and other explorers have reported similar sightings. If you stay awake, when you witness the glory of nature, you can too. We all have the ability to communicate on a very deep level with nature. It is an expression of the same energy that created us. Ultimately, we are one.

Experience the Movie of Life

We may all be watching a movie on the ABC TV Channel in America, and we may think the story is the best reflection of our own lives, but all we have to do is switch over to the CBS channel, and we will encounter a completely different story. NBC is a whole different world too. Then we switch over to HBO or the BBC, and you get the idea. The Universe is like that. There are infinite channels or frequencies of life. We are only aware of the one we are currently living and awake to.

As we become awake to our deep natural awareness, we will start to experience other frequencies. Most people see in color, but some people have a monochromatic vision and only see in black and white. There are many frequencies representing different colors and sounds, some we can see and hear others we can't. We only use a very small percentage of our brain, but we have the innate propensity to experience much more than we are currently aware of.

During the seventies, the Central Intelligence Agency (CIA) commissioned a group of people, who had clairvoyant abilities to spy on Russian intercontinental ballistic missile (ICBM) sites, by using what they called a Remote Viewing technique. It ended up being called the Stargate Project. The group would sit in a building outside of Stanford University, meditate for a while and try to picture the map coordinates of Russian ICBM sites. Apparently, the Russians had a similar program.

They actually had enough success that they continued studying the process for several years. A funny movie about the CIA Remote Viewing program was released in 2009, *The Men Who Stare at Goats,* starring Ewan McGregor. The movie was a comedy, but the core of the story was true. The CIA really did spend more than $20 million, and several years studying the process.

You don't have to be in your body with your eyes open to see. When we dream at night, our eyes are shut, but we still see, and some people, including myself, have actually had out-of-body, or near-death experiences where we see clearly while not even being in our bodies. Seeing, like feeling and hearing, is just a state of awareness. It may be hard to comprehend, but if you have experienced it, you will understand. We all have the ability to experience different dimensions of reality, not just clairvoyant psychics recruited by the CIA.

Experience the God Test

Pythagoras figured out a whole language using numerology thousands of years ago. He developed his own intricate system of numbers that guide the direction of your life, and if you believe in it, it will start to work for you. However, you can also develop your own system, and if you believe in it, it will work too. The number seventy-seven has serendipitously come up repeatedly at auspicious times throughout my life so once in a playful test to myself, I asked God to show himself to me by showing me the number seventy-seven. Wherever I go, I now constantly see the number seventy-seven on license plates, billboards, magazine covers, road signs, the Internet, and TV. The number pops up everywhere.

Try it for yourself. It doesn't necessarily have to be the number seventy-seven, it can be any number, just as your name for God can be any name, and it will still work. What is your favorite number? Give it a try. Don't think it is hard enough? Then use a combination of your favorite numbers. You will soon realize it is beyond normal logic or statistical analysis how often the specific combination of numbers shows up in your life.

You will soon realize the truth; God always surrounds you, and is always part of you, because Being is God. When you are awake to your union with Being, you are controlling your own destiny, and if you decide God is represented by a certain number or combination of numbers that is what you will experience.

Experience Ego Versus Being

Imagine you are a twin separated at birth from your identical brother. Your parents were briefly in love but soon started fighting, quickly divorced, swore never to speak again, and moved to different cities. You and your identical brother have never spoken. You didn't even know the other existed. Since your parents resented each other so much, they both agreed to never even mention the other again.

Your mother moved to San Francisco with your brother, and you moved with your father to Los Angeles. Your father had flamboyant Italian ancestry, and he was a Ferrari mechanic. Since

Step Five: EXPERIENCE

you grew up surrounded by Ferraris, you totally appreciated their fine craftsmanship, high style, and speed. You worked hard in your father's garage, and when you were sixteen, your father fixed up an old Ferrari and gave it to you.

Your identical twin brother grew up with your mom in San Francisco. He followed her compassionate Irish nature, and he eventually started working alongside her as a photographer at the Sierra Club. Your mom was so proud of your brother when he turned sixteen she bought him a silver, hybrid Toyota Prius.

One day you take your Ferrari up the coast from LA to Big Sur where the winding roads are perfect for racing your Ferrari at top speed. Your identical brother is driving down the coast in his Prius to photograph the magnificent nature of Big Sur like his hero, Ansel Adams. Your brother had traveled all the way down the coast that morning at sunrise to photograph the sun shining out across the ocean. Now he is looking for a place to turn around to head back north, up the coast to San Francisco.

You come speeding around the corner, headed north in your Ferrari with loud music blaring, enjoying every fast turn, and you see this silver Prius ahead of you do a U-turn right in front of you. You almost hit him, but since your bloodline traces back to the racing legend, Mario Andretti, you downshift, and brake expertly to miss the collision. You are furious because this imbecile, driving the Prius, almost killed you.

Now as you follow him, heading north up the coast, you are forced to drive the exact speed limit. You can't pass him on the narrow winding road with oncoming traffic, and you get more and more frustrated until you are about to explode. These are the kind of people you can't stand – self-righteous, Prius driving, do-gooders that have missed the point of life – to have fun and to live to the fullest! Your identical brother, meanwhile, sees your Ferrari in his rearview mirror, tailgating him, constantly trying to pass, and he detests you. You are exactly what is wrong with the world today – a narcissistic, rich, gas guzzling, Ferrari driving, polluter.

The slow Prius, crawling along in front of you, is making you livid. You see your chance to pass. You know you have the speed to do it, so you go for it. Your brother watches you make the idiotic move of passing him right before the turn, and he can't believe it.

As you pass him, he flips you the bird, and everything goes into slow motion, as you look across to see your identical twin for the first time. It is *you* driving the Prius. His mouth drops open, as he realizes it is *him* driving the Ferrari. You hear a loud horn, and you look up to see an oncoming truck. You turn hard left to avoid the head-on crash, but you hit the Prius, and both of your cars tumble off the cliff. You crash on the rocks, a hundred feet below – both cars explode, and you both die.

When you meet in heaven you don't need to talk, you both immediately know what your life lesson was – you are one and the same. We are all one and the same. We are not a Ferrari or a Prius. Those are the ego created vehicles, our bodies, in which we travel through life. We are not black people and white people; we are not Chinese, Americans, Russians, Israelis, or Iranians – we are each souls, Beings, all from the same Source, only traveling in different, unique bodies. We must begin to recognize and identify with that truth before we crash. *Breathe and Accept the Now; Feel and Experience Being Awareness.*

Chapter Six

Step Six
BEING

Accept the feeling you are having right now, transcend every desire, transcend all thoughts, and feel your experience transform into the silent peace of Being. Just be. Do nothing else. Just be. *Become aware you are an expression of the Source of all creation, Being, and identify yourself with that experience.* Being is naturally the state of deep, fulfilling, profound peace, and the more you become aware of that; the more you will experience it.

Identifying with your ego is the biggest obstacle to enlightenment. Your ego is leading you on its own course, and that course can be in the exact opposite direction of the experience of Being. You must redirect your awareness to experience Being.

Experience your Higher Self more and more, and your lower self will fade into the background. It is imperative to always remember *Being is always there at the core of your existence.* No matter how depressed you presently feel emotionally, always remember Being is always simultaneously there in the background. You only have to shift your awareness to it in order to start experiencing it.

Witness your misguided ego and the games it plays. Don't give your ego any power, and it will subside to the point it will eventually start leading you in the direction of Being. Your ego will always be there even when you are enlightened, but it will slip into the background. You will be lead instead by Being. Allow Being to become the prominent experience in your life.

Being Attracts Being

As you put more attention to your awareness, the experience of Being will attract more of the experience of Being. All states of consciousness perpetuate similar states of consciousness. The experience of Being becomes deeper and more profound as we become more awake to the infinite possibilities of Being.

Being becomes easier to access and to enjoy, the more you are able to experience it. It feels like a snowball rolling down a hill getting bigger and bigger. The laughter, happiness, and joy continue to increase while the feeling of deep peace and contentment is always there at the core. Once Being has been experienced for an extended period, everything else becomes less crucial. However, you don't withdraw from life; instead, you find everything in life so much more fun and fulfilling.

Believe in Being

When I was a kid, whenever we went to church at the end of every sermon we repeated the word, "Amen," like parrots, but we never really knew what the word meant. Twenty years later at my older brother's wedding, the pastor informed us the interpretation of Amen from ancient Hebrew is: "I believe it will be so." In the Bible, Jesus said, "All things are possible for one who believes."[10]

In chapter one, I told you the story of how late in 2007, I

Step Six: BEING

directed Kobe Bryant in a Public Service Announcement that ended up being broadcast on TV in 2008, to put attention on the atrocities occurring in Darfur. When I met Kobe, I was in awe of the great confidence that emanated from him. I said, "Kobe, you embody a sense of pure confidence. You remind me of one of those Spartan warriors from the movie, *300*." He laughed, and replied, "Yeah, we watch that movie all the time." I shared his laugh, but it wasn't until I read his great coach, Phil Jackson's book, *Sacred Hoops*, I totally understood what he meant. Kobe watched the movie, *300*, because it was part of his game plan for achieving success.

In the movie, *300*, a group of 300 Spartan warriors defeats a million Persian soldiers, only because they truly believed they could. Their incredible belief in themselves was the key to victory. Kobe watched the movie as a placebo effect to instill belief in himself. It is easy to understand when you step onto the national stage and play basketball in front of millions of people it must be terrifying unless you are able to harness enormous confidence. To gain confidence, you need belief. You see where you want the ball to go, take a deep breath, shoot, and because you totally believe it is going in, it does.

It is not an accident the Lakers under the coaching of Phil Jackson won five NBA championships, and Jackson won six NBA titles previously, coaching the Chicago Bulls. The combination of visionary coaches like Phil Jackson and enormously talented players like Kobe Bryant, and Michael Jordan, that truly understand the whole game, not just the physical game, made teams like the Lakers and the Bulls big winners.

Believing in, and then experiencing Being is the key to any success in life. It is the key to any creation, but truly believing is a lot more difficult than most "Law of Attraction" based books would have you have you think. Your experience will quickly teach you how difficult it is to truly believe in your ability to create. Chant to yourself all day long, write pictures on your mirror, the wall, the ceiling above your bed, tattoo it to your arm, talk yourself into it as much as you can, but your chances are still next to none you are going to win the Lotto. If it were easy, we'd all be super rich.

Once, when my son was a very little boy, I was driving back to Los Angeles with my wife and son from a Christmas ski vacation in Telluride, Colorado. We left Telluride on New Year's day, early in the morning, with only half a tank of gas because the station in town was still closed when we left. We had been hit by a huge snowstorm, and it had snowed every day the previous week. While that had been great for powder skiing, it was a major impediment to the journey home. My Jeep was covered in about two feet of snow, and like a bad Boy Scout, I never prepared properly for the road trip home by filling my gas tank the day before when the gas stations were open.

That mistake was compounded by the fact that instead of leaving the town by our usual route, going over the back mountain pass, headed southwest toward Arizona, which I concluded was too deep in snow to cross, we headed northwest toward Utah, which I had never done before. I was not relying on an actual GPS, but a *Map Blast* map I had printed from the Internet the night before. My final mistake was this northern route home to Los Angeles would take us right through Las Vegas, and I wanted to stop there for the night which is, admittedly, a crazy incentive to head out across uncharted land on New Year's day in the deep snow with half a tank of gas.

We had been traveling on local roads across vast fields of snow without sight of civilization for several hours when I started to get a little bit nervous. The gas tank had been on empty for a few miles, and my old Blackberry was getting no signal. We had no actual map of the area and not a clue where the next gas station was. I looked in the backseat at my little son,

Step Six: BEING

Weston, buckled into his jump seat, and I started to feel like a total fool. I should've known better than this. I grew up skiing in the mountains. Now, being a total idiot, I was going to have to flag down a cowboy, and beg for some gas, or else we were going to freeze to death.

I took several deep breaths. I totally accepted my situation. I felt the presence of exactly that moment, and I was aware of the feeling of Being. I appreciated my beautiful wife, child, and everything I could see in front of me, and I totally *believed* we were going to be all right. Sure enough, we traveled another mile, completely riding on fumes, and there was a gas station. By the grace of God, it was open on New Year's day.

Not impressed? It gets better. Here's the end of the story, which brings us back to hitting the Lotto and creating wealth by completely believing in Being. We get to Vegas. My wife is not happy. We had spent the previous week in beautiful Telluride, Colorado, surrounded by Mother Nature. Every falling snowflake was a testimony to the greatness of God, and here we were driving at night into a neon jungle full of decadence and debauchery. I still was glad we were there. Yes, it is a different channel, a different frequency of energy, but it can be a lot of fun if you can escape judgmental mode. Sheila is not very judgmental, but instinctively she knew better than I that Las Vegas is not the best place to bring a little boy. After reaching our hotel room I agreed to leave the next morning, but first I wanted to play one fast hand of blackjack.

I awoke early the next morning and started to meditate. While my wife and son slept, I meditated for an hour and a half. They awoke, and they went downstairs for breakfast. I continued to meditate. I had promised Sheila I was only going to play one fast hand of blackjack, and I was only going to bet a very small amount, twenty dollars. Win or lose I would quit after that, but my plan was a little more devious – I was conspiring with the

Source to win. I had been meditating for over thirty-five years. If I couldn't create one very small win in Vegas, then this whole "believing" concept doesn't really work. I meditated even longer. After two hours of meditation, I went downstairs to the large casino on the first floor. I bought twenty dollars worth of chips, walked up to the first blackjack table, bet all my chips, and I swear to almighty God, I got an ace and a jack with my first two cards – Blackjack. I more than doubled my money, and I left the table to have breakfast with my family.

Okay, I know what you're thinking. If I can do that with only twenty dollars, why not up the ante, and make thousands? And if it really works, why don't I make millions? All I can say is, yes, theoretically that works too, but no, I can't guarantee I can do it. Why not? I proved I could do it. Yes, that was with twenty dollars. Up the stakes to a hundred, I can probably still pull it off. However, if you up the stakes to a thousand, and one thought of doubt creeps in, because a thousand dollars is a lot to lose, and that one doubtful thought changes the order sent to the Source; failure can easily be the outcome.

So the question is, do I want to spend two hours each morning in Las Vegas meditating in order to make twenty dollars? No, the math doesn't work, that won't even pay for breakfast.

So now the final question is – how does Kobe, or Michael Jordan or any other major winner do it with so much on the line? They don't. Not all of the time. They just do it more than anyone else. Even superstars have their periods in the Zone, and their periods out of the Zone. The good news for you is the Seven Steps will help put you in the Zone, more and more, and the creation of your desires will definitely reflect that. However, there is one big caveat – your desires to get rich and famous are generated by your ego, and your ego has a lot less power to create. Being can create anything, instantly, but Being doesn't necessarily want to become rich and famous. Being doesn't need to be rich and famous to feel completely content and loved. Being is already absolutely content. Being is pure love.

Totally Believing in Being is a Feeling

According to the New Oxford American Dictionary: believe, means: *accept* (something) as true; *feel* sure of the veracity of.

If you are not totally sure something is going to happen, it won't. You have to completely believe, but once you totally believe it will happen, it will. You have to believe it to the point you can *feel* something will happen. When you actually can *feel* it is going to happen, it absolutely, most definitely, will.

The Force is With You

In December 2017, Star Wars broke box office records again with its sequel: *Star Wars: The Last Jedi*. I saw the movie at the Director's Guild of America (DGA) with my 15-year-old son, Weston, and his friend. Both boys are huge Star Wars fans. At lunch afterwards, it was immediately apparent they both had a much vaster knowledge than I did about the Star Wars plot line and the characters, even though the original Star Wars was more in line with my generation than theirs. The details get a little confusing unless you've really paid attention to all eight of the Star Wars movies over the past forty years.

My son and his friend are Star Wars fans with tons of knowledge, and they had fun ridiculing my lack of Star Wars trivia. Even on a more profound level, they intuitively were deeply attracted to Star Wars. Inherently, my son and his friend, like millions of fans across planet Earth, are deeply attracted to Star Wars because it is modern mythology dealing with our innate connection to The Force.

The Force is not just some contrived storyline that sounds clever. George Lucas had explained Zen Buddhism was a major influence when he wrote the original Star Wars. He may have created his own version of how The Force works, but at its core a lot of it is true.

Other extremely successful movies, like *The Matrix, Harry Potter, and Dr. Strange* have tapped into the same concept from totally different perspectives. Why are these movies so incredibly successful? Because they tune into our innate curiosity about tapping into a force that can make each of us superstars.

We all want to be a Jedi Knight. We all want to be Superman. We all want superpowers, and that is because we each have the natural ability to actually gain superpowers. I know it sounds like preposterous science fiction, but some unique people (and all of us to a lesser degree) have performed miracles throughout time. There are amazing stories of special gurus in India that have been able to move small objects with their thoughts. Is it true? Well, maybe not at the level we see in movies, but you will just have to start exploring yourself and see what your experience teaches you. I believe anything is possible if we truly believe in Being. *Breathe and Accept the Now; Feel and Experience Being Awareness.*

Chapter Seven

Step Seven
AWARENESS

Being Awareness

Your Higher Self, experiencing Being, is Being Awareness. Your Higher Self is your individual soul. Your soul is your individual awareness of Being. Your individual awareness is experiencing whole, absolute Being. Your Higher Self, individual awareness, is experiencing the infinite, eternal Source. *God is experiencing God.* Being Awareness is the final step. Initially, this concept is abstract and hard to comprehend, however, through experience it will become clear. Enlightenment is becoming awake to the continual *Experience of Being Awareness.*

Transcend All Desires to Experience Being Awareness

The experience of Being Awareness can only continue to be maintained when you have transcended all desires. Accept everything the way it is. Accept the Now. Feel it. Experience it. Be Aware of Being.

Awareness is the Final Step

The Seven Steps become one step – Awareness. Simple, effortless, innocent, transcendental Awareness is Being Awareness. Being Awareness is the final step to experiencing the peace, love, happiness, and bliss of enlightenment. Breathing, Accepting Now, Feeling, and Experiencing Being, are the first six essential steps that allow you to experience the absolute peace of Being, but the final step, to *remain Aware of the experience of Being*, is what allows love, happiness, and bliss to become your reality. Being Awareness is the catalyst that allows the ultimate, blissful feeling of enlightenment to be experienced. We can walk into a dark forest at night, and it may be the same forest, but it is not until the sun lights it up that we are able to see its beauty. The first six Essential Steps are the forest; the Seventh Step, Awareness, is the light.

The experience of Being Awareness results in the experience of bliss. Refined happiness, bliss, is the ultimate expression of the absolute peace of Being as it manifests in the relative world. Being is God. *God's direct expression in the relative world is peace, love, happiness, and bliss. Through the Experience of Being Awareness, you will feel universal love, happiness, and bliss.*

Put it to the test. Let your experience teach you. Sit alone in a room. Experiencing Being Awareness doesn't preclude interacting with other people, but it is easier, in the beginning to be alone without any obvious distractions. Take a deep breath, and accept anything that comes your way. Feel the very subtle feeling of nothingness behind everything. Feel the absolute silence of Being behind any sounds in the room. Now effortlessly become aware of it. As you effortlessly become aware of the absolute silence as the Source of everything, Being instantly becomes a beautiful, transcendent feeling of peace, love, and happiness.

As you now look around the room, and innocently are aware of it, accepting everything, you will become aware of the intrinsic beauty of a window in the corner of the room letting in the sunshine. Your guitar leaning against the wall, calling to be played. The bookcase with rows of books containing stories you absolutely love. All the material objects in the room will come to life with love. You will feel the absolute peace behind everything. *Be aware of Being as the Source of everything you encounter in life; peace, love, happiness, and bliss will be your experience.*

Awareness of the Glow

The actual experience of Being Awareness will be very subtle at first, sometimes so subtle you won't be aware of it at all. You have to understand the Source, Being, is not here in the relative world we live in. It is beyond this world in the infinite, absolute world. It is the Source of everything in our relative existence, but it is not actually in the relative world we live in. It is beyond us.

However, if we broaden our awareness by transcending thinking, then we will be aware of Being in the background, behind everything, as the Source of everything. If we put our attention on it and stay aware of it, the feeling will glow. The feeling of glowing will be an obvious, tangible feeling of profound peace, love, happiness, and bliss.

Feel the energy in your body change. Be aware of that feeling, and more of that peaceful feeling of love, happiness, and bliss will come. The awareness of the feeling of Being is attracting more of itself. Feelings are vibrations, and all vibrations attract similar vibrations. *Remember, practicing Being Awareness is the most essential step to experiencing the peace, love, happiness, and bliss of enlightenment.* Practice it, and your experience will teach you it works. Then do it again, and again, until it becomes a natural, automatic, effortless habit.

Being Awareness Leads to Unity Consciousness

When you start seeing life through the eyes of someone who is in a state of what I call "Being Awareness," it is contagious. Being

Awareness attracts more awareness of Being; love attracts more love until that is all you see. When you reach that point, you have entered the world of Unity Consciousness, where everywhere you look you see a reflection of the love you are projecting. You are seeing life through the eyes of God. God loves everyone and everything. I know it sounds absolutely fantastic and too good to be true, but in small examples, I am sure you have already experienced it.

Maybe you have experienced a taste of Unity Consciousness at your best friends wedding where everyone loves the new bride, and groom, including you, and all of their friends instantly become your new friends. The wedding is absolutely phenomenal, under a big white tent in the middle of a beautiful field, and the band is playing some fantastic music everybody just loves dancing to. It feels like every partner you dance with, you want to marry. That is a taste of Unity Consciousness. There is no judgment, no separation, and no thoughts, just laughing, and dancing. Life can actually be like that the majority of the time.

Accept Being Awareness

Take a deep breath, and accept what you are feeling, hearing, experiencing, right now, even if it is background noise you initially have an aversion to. Just accept it, feel and experience Being behind the sound, at the source of the sound. Now be *aware of* that experience of Being, and you will notice the sound will change. It will become more soothing, peaceful, and happy. *Always remember you are an expression of Being, God, already totally connected to Being.* Be Aware of that reality, and your experience of peace, love, happiness, and bliss will confirm you are on the right track to enlightenment. Become aware of the very subtle feeling of Being, and you will automatically smile and feel at peace. Being is the absolute peace of nothingness

Step Seven: AWARENESS

behind everything. Being is the absolute Source of everything; Being is omnipresent latent potential. *Being Awareness allows Being to come alive in our relative world as peace, love, happiness, and bliss. Breathe and Accept the Now; Feel and Experience Being Awareness.*

Chapter Eight

THE SEVEN STEPS

Why the Seven Steps?

I had exclusively been practicing Vedic mantra-based meditation (TM) for 40 years, and it worked well. However, I wanted a technique in addition to Vedic mantra meditation I could practice twenty-four hours a day, seven days a week. I didn't want to only meditate in the morning for twenty minutes, or even several hours, and then again in the evening. I didn't want to only meditate for a limited amount of time, then go out into the day, and slowly fall back into the world that my ego created, when that world still lacked in so many ways. I asked God for guidance; the Seven Steps of the BANFEBA Meditation technique were the answer.

Once you understand how incredible life can be when your awareness is expanded, once you have had a taste of enlightenment, you want more. You want to live it every day, all day long. BANFEBA Meditation will allow you to do that. BANFEBA Meditation is a technique that will allow you to expedite your journey to experience an enlightened life of peace, love, happiness, and bliss.

I created the Seven Steps of the BANFEBA Meditation as my personal technique to reach enlightenment faster. Then as I would spontaneously meet people, who were also on a similar spiritual path, I would feel the connection, and I would automatically start teaching what they inherently wanted to know. The Universe was constantly connecting me with people similar to myself that had tasted the fine nectar of enlightenment and desperately craved more. I also profoundly wanted to leave my son, Weston, all the knowledge I had learned in this lifetime. I wanted to give Weston, and all beings on Earth, peace, love, and happiness. That's when I decided to write this book.

Suggestions as You Practice the Seven Steps

Very few spiritual books or teachers talk about the possible negative side effects of trying to reach enlightenment. It is always good to stay positive and not put any attention on the negative aspects of life, or those negative aspects will grow. Whatever you predominately think and feel will attract similar thoughts and feelings until those feelings will become the dominant reality you experience as your life.

The good side of that equation is when you use the Seven Steps to eventually transcend the mind and completely become aware of your connection with Being, you will be immersing yourself in absolute peace, love, happiness, and bliss, and it is so powerful, nothing can pull you away from that feeling for very long. The only caveat is – the road getting to this blissful place is not always smooth.

Speed Bumps

When you practice the Seven Steps, you will experience an expanded state of awareness, and you will begin to experience feelings most other people are not awake to. You will become very sensitive to everything around you. At first, it will take time to synthesize this new reality. You will also have access to much more energy to create your reality faster than you ever had before. That infinite energy has always been there, but now you are finally aware of it, and you are now able to tap into it.

Most people walk down the road of life. They are going slow enough so if they get off the path and bump into a tree, it won't hurt much because they are moving so slowly. However, when you are experiencing a state of higher consciousness, you are moving down the road much faster. You're not walking anymore; you're driving. Eventually, you're not driving slowly. You're driving fast, very fast, until the point you feel like you're driving on the Swiss Autobahn in a Lamborghini. So now when you drive fast off the path, which in the beginning is inevitable because you still need to learn the skills to maintain proper navigation – you will tumble through the air, cartwheeling past trees. It can be very unsettling, even do damage, and if you hit a tree, it can be totally destructive.

Your actual experience will vary, but it may include periods of anger, doubt, anxiety, insecurity, frustration, and unhappiness. The reason for this is your awareness is fluctuating between awareness of Being – peace, love, happiness, and bliss – to normal, mind-dominated, dysfunction of thinking. This new awakened perspective will make that old dysfunction now seem almost unbearable. The good news is this is only a stage, and you will eventually pass through it. Your awareness is becoming awake to your ego's control and putting it into its proper perspective. Ultimately, this is a good thing.

Ego Traps

Your ego naturally wants to own any experience you create and take full credit for it. Ironically, your identification with the ego will stop the creative process. The closer you get to enlightenment, the easier it is to fall into this trap. Your ego becomes big, to stay in control, to fight off the infinite power of Being that you are now becoming aware of.

The key is not to fight your ego but to *accept* it, to transcend it, and experience Being. All of my personal life stories, including some that I've mentioned here, were teaching me that lesson in one way or another. Look at your own life, and you will see your life stories are also teaching you the same lesson in different ways.

The expanding ego is a clever trap for spiritual seekers at all levels of experience, and if you look carefully, you will see some disingenuous gurus and spiritual teachers that have imploded during the process. They start acting condescending and superior – a few even proclaiming to be God. A grain of sand is part of the beach, and that connection will allow it to experience being the whole beach, but just because that grain of sand rides a wave out to sea, it doesn't mean the whole beach is going to follow it.

Keep an eye on your own experiences, and the world you are beginning to create, and always be ready to jump back into the safety net of your natural connection with Being. When you are aware of your innate connection with Being nothing can stop you or hurt you – you are invincible – but as soon as you let your ego subdue your awareness of Being, you will be back, alone, fighting the world you have created, only now because your ego is bigger, your world is even bigger. When you read these words you may want to get off this path, thinking to yourself, life is okay now simply walking through it; I don't really need a Lamborghini to go so fast.

So this is where we leave the imperfect analogy, and jump back to the truth no one can escape – you don't have a choice. We are all on the same path. We are all on the path to enlightenment whether we know it or not, and whether we like it or not. So we all have to go through this process. The only choice is when. *If you are reading this now, then now is the time for you.* There are no accidents in life. You have created everything in your existence down to the smallest details, relationships, and events.

It is all your creation. You hearing these words is your creation. You have asked your Self, Being, the question, and Being is now answering. If you don't like this particular answer, Being will answer in a different way through another person, book, or event, but ultimately the answer is all the same, just told in a myriad of different ways. The answer is *you are on the path to enlightenment.*

My advice is don't worry about the speed bumps, you will get over them, you will miss the trees, you will have a lot of fun on your journey, and you will reach enlightenment. *The trees and the speed bumps are only there to keep us on track. Accept the obstacles. Learn from them.* When you realize you have diverted off course, use the Seven Steps to get back on the path.

Remember to Accept Your Ego to Transcend it

When you become belligerent, or contentious, when you defend yourself in an argument, when you brag, when you fantasize, when you daydream, when you judge anyone or anything in any manner, when you fight to make a point, when you try to stand up for what is right, when you are proud – that is all your ego creating your reality. If you exclusively attach yourself to that reality, you are setting yourself up for defeat, sorrow, and unhappiness. When you have an unending chain of desires – you are only identifying with your lower self, your ego. You need to use the Seven Steps to transcend your desires, transcend thinking, and experience Being, so none of these traps have any power over you.

Once you continually experience Being, you will be able to witness your thinking mind, without being taken over by it. You still may act in any of the ways mentioned above, but you will not be caught in the trap. You will be able to transcend the chain of thoughts at any time and experience the peace, love, happiness, and bliss of Being.

The Seven Steps and Religion

The wonderful part of organized religion is everyone gets dressed up, puts on their best face, greets others with respect, and understands they are part of a great mission to search for God. All of that, plus singing, meeting new friends, and building a healthy community are positive influences in our lives. If you are now part of any organized religion, please stick with it if you have positive experiences. The Seven Steps will allow you to appreciate those positive experiences even more.

The challenging part of organized religion is it sometimes separates us into camps, where we end up becoming self-righteous and judgmental. Or we are reminded of how we have been "bad" in the past, and we feel guilty. Religion also sometimes feels hard to relate to because we are telling stories that are so old, they have very little relevance to our own contemporary lives.

The extreme misinterpretation of religion is when we totally believe in God, and our connection to God, and then we believe our special path to God is so perfect all other paths are completely wrong. We believe we are the chosen ones, and we are willing to die to do what we think is God's work here on Earth. All we have to do is tune into any news channel, or website, to see the fanatical aspects of religion, where people are blowing themselves, and other people, up as a vindication of their religious beliefs.

Many in the world, especially in America, are now turning their backs on organized religion because of this fanatical extremism, but as we get older, there is always something pulling us back. That is our own inherent connection with Being. We innately know there is something missing in our lives, and we are all looking for it. At the core of each major religion practiced in the world today, there is a spiritual truth that although it may be hard to understand, always pulls us back. If you are an Atheist and want absolutely no connection to the word God, I recommend you invent your own vocabulary. Call it anything that works for you, but keep using the Seven Steps to allow the experience of a higher state of consciousness to become a reality in your life. Enlightenment, Unity Consciousness, or whatever you want to call it, is your destiny. Let your experience be your teacher.

Astrology / Jyotish / Numerology / Psychics

As we use the Seven Steps to reach higher states of consciousness sometimes, it is easy to get sidetracked. We are all curious about our future, and we are always looking for advice on how to get what we desire in life. In every city across the country, and around the world, there are plenty of astrologers, numerologists, tarot card readers, Jyotish masters, and psychics, who for a price will show us the way. Sometimes, they can give us good advice, teach us that everything in the Universe is interconnected, and prove to us the theory behind their particular craft has validity. But we must beware – many of them only have a rudimentary knowledge of their craft, and they can lead us into trouble.

They tell us something about our future, we believe them, and then that event transpires, but it happens only because we believe it. What happens if they tell us something catastrophic? The placebo effect is very powerful. We can't let someone else control our destiny. We must always remember. We are in control. We are a lot more powerful than some cards, or the date we were born on. They may tap into a view of what we have created so far in life, but we must always remember – *we have the power to change our future at any point.*

One time someone asked Maharishi if some psychics could actually communicate with, and get advice from, the dead? And apparently, Maharishi characteristically laughed, and responded, "Yes, sometimes they can, but just because they are dead doesn't mean they are right!"

During the eighties there was a rumor that circulated in America – First Lady, Nancy Reagan, was apparently seeing an astrologer and then advising her husband, President Reagan. I remember thinking that's kind of a scary thought, isn't it? Should we invade Panama? Not sure, let's see what the cards say. I also heard intriguing stories about investment bankers and traders on Wall Street in New York City that made fortunes off of tips from their psychics, but I would always think if it really works, why aren't the psychics themselves getting extremely rich?

One time, while living in New York City, I heard about this prominent psychic several movie stars would consult. I was curious, looking for answers on when I was going to be able to launch my first movie, so I visited this famous psychic, hoping she was one of the few psychics that actually are clairvoyant. Before I arrived, I had just finished my extensive, two-hour mediation program, and I was feeling fantastic.

I entered through the door and walked into her apartment. She looked at me with eyes wide open, and she literally gasped. She said, "I see a large aura of white light coming from your head. You are connected to God. You are directly connected to Jesus." Then she said something that literally sent shivers up my spine. She said, "In your last life, you were one of the Disciples of Christ."

She wasn't sure which one I was, but she was totally convinced about the Jesus connection. This meeting with the famous psychic happened before my visit from Jesus, so I had no indication if she was right, but of course, my ego loved to hear it. On the way home, I couldn't stop thinking about it. As I mentioned earlier, I did not grow up in a very religious family, and I spent very little time studying *The Bible,* so I walked into the nearest bookstore, and I started reading everything I could on the Disciples of Jesus.

Is it true? Who knows? Is anything said by a psychic true? Sure, some of it is, but I believe the only way anyone should take anything seriously is by putting it through the filter of his or her own experience. Experience is what teaches.

Several years later, I was living in Los Angeles, and an older, meditating friend, mentioned he knew of this psychic that was completely crazy, but extremely accurate. So, again, I wanted to see when I was going to launch my second movie, so I went to see her.

When I entered her house, I realized this lady is perfect casting for the crazy psychic lady. She weighed about three hundred pounds, and she had a posse of cats surrounding her. Her small house was full of crystals, statues of Hindu and Buddhist Deities, and she had lit candles everywhere.

I walked up the cramped stairs, entered a dark room, and I saw her sitting, meditating, in a trance in front of her crystals. She kept her eyes closed as I mumbled a greeting, and she smiled as I sat down. I don't remember anything from our brief conversation except when our eyes finally connected, she looked straight at me, and said, "In your last life, you were a Disciple of Christ. You were St Bartholomew."

Ego Traps Can Dominate Your Experience of Life

Always remember, as you use the Seven Steps to reach a state of higher consciousness, if you don't stay perfectly balanced, the ego will set traps for you. Whatever gets you thinking in cycles, controls you – even if it is true. If it is a compelling fantasy or even an attractive real story you continually tell yourself, then the ego always goes to it. That is a trap.

As your presence grows, and you tap into expanded awareness, your dreams and fantasies will come to life in a big way. It is ironic because the more enlightened you become, the more you will be able to create your reality according to your fantasies of greatness, but those new realities of greatness will have a bigger ability for your ego to trap you. A lot of my personal life stories on my spiritual journey are a good example of that.

All of the famous people I have met in life, some of whom I mention in this book, are an example of our ability to create our own reality based on our desires as we expand our awareness of Being. As I became more awake, I would naturally meet them because at some point I wished I would. I drop their names because they are famous, so they are easy to track. I hope it proves the point, and the stories are fun. It is fun to create an exciting reality, but we must always be on guard because it can be a trap. Our egos love it, but we must be careful. We can all enjoy our exciting new realities, but we must transcend all desires to maintain our awareness of Being. Stay awake to Being, and realize Being is the source of our exciting new realities. Being is what allows our dreams to become our reality.

Awareness Comes in Stages

The Universe is infinitely powerful, and when you connect with it using the Seven Steps, you have the ability to integrate perfectly with that power – but you have to be careful, because you are still operating out of your human body, and it can only handle so much energy at different stages of your awareness.

Think of an extremely powerful light socket with a bulb that can only handle so much wattage. If you are not careful, you can burn out the light bulb. Eventually, through your identification with Being, by continually practicing the Seven Steps, you will be able to handle more and more energy, but it comes in incremental stages of increased awareness.

Subliminal Communication

As your consciousness becomes more awake, continually using the Seven Steps, you will begin to realize the majority of our communication in life with other human beings is subliminal. Everyone already does this, but we are mostly unaware of the process.

Before we start talking to someone, we have already communicated a lot of information subliminally. We have already assessed that person's general personality traits. We already understand a lot about that person. As we become extremely awake, we feel the Source of another person's thoughts because it is the Source of our thoughts too, and if we are aware enough, we can actually hear their thoughts. At first, it is mostly a feeling, but I believe the process has the ability to become very clear, where you can hear the actual words.

When Jesus visited me, his thoughts were loud and clear like an actual voice. That was an extremely unique experience, but I believe as a species we will all eventually evolve to the point where we can clearly hear each other's thoughts, and there will be less need for verbal communication. This will be a great stage of evolution because when we are awake enough to actually hear each other's thoughts we will also be awake enough to recognize our unity as human beings, and there will be no more wars or fighting.

Subliminal communication can happen in mundane, ordinary communication with your friends, family, or even strangers too, where you can begin to hear the feelings or emotions of another, but it is usually not as obvious because we are not as awake to the experience. Special encounters with important people encourage us to be more observant, and we sometimes have the opportunity to notice subliminal communication more.

When I met Barack Obama, I remember very clearly the encounter. It was at the presidential election caucus in 2008, in the afternoon, in a large school gym, in the snowy fields of Iowa. Iowa is the first caucus; therefore, it is important to win there in a presidential election because it gives the candidates enormous momentum as they then head for the New Hampshire primary.

I was filming from the stage where the press were designated to shoot from, directly opposite the stage where Senator Obama was giving a speech. As I listened to the speech while looking through the viewfinder of my camera, I felt this enormous connection with Obama. I had seen his campaign bus parked next to our film bus, as we traveled across Iowa to shoot our documentary, several times over the past week. For some serendipitous reason we always linked up and ended up in the same parking lot of the same hotel, parked next to each other, and I was very curious about this African American presidential candidate.

By that point in the week of traveling across the state I had filmed and met most of the candidates, and when I separated them from their politics, I liked most of them because of their very interesting personalities. Bill Clinton was extremely intelligent with an enormous amount of charisma. Hillary Clinton was also very intelligent, and she was extremely well prepared. John McCain was a great storyteller. It was obvious to me Mitt Romney was on a deep spiritual mission, and I was able to talk to him personally for about ten minutes, but it was not his time to be president. I met the other candidates too, but they didn't make as strong of an impression.

As I listened to Obama that day in Iowa, I was so incredibly inspired, because he was very intelligent like Bill Clinton. He had a strong spiritual connection like Mitt Romney. He had a great sense of humor like John F Kennedy. And his most valuable characteristic as a politician was he could inspire as he spoke like Dr. Martin Luther King, Jr. It was an unbeatable combination. I thought to myself, wow, this guy could really be the first African American president of the United States of America. It was a very exciting, auspicious place and time, and I felt everyone else in the room felt that excitement too.

After Obama spoke, he moved along the edge of the stage, and he started shaking hands with people in the crowd. I quickly grabbed my camera. I jumped off the press stage, and I worked my way across the sea of people to the stage where Obama had been speaking. For some reason, I really wanted to meet him personally and shake his hand too. As a member of the press that is not really the proper protocol, but I didn't care. I just wanted to meet this guy.

Now you have to remember at that particular time in 2008, at the launch of the presidential race, Obama was a complete underdog. Yes, a lot of other political pundits recognized his star potential too, but I am not sure many people thought it was totally possible in America to break that cultural, racial barrier, yet.

I was navigating my way through the crowd, as it was breaking up. Most people were now headed for the doors. I kept my eye on Obama, and I was slightly disappointed because he was moving away from me toward the side of the stage to the exit, shaking hands along the way. I thought that's a drag, he's going to escape out the side, and I'm not going to be able to meet him. Then something very strange happened. Obama looked out into the dispersing crowd on the basketball court, and he saw me fighting the crowd to get to him, our eyes locked, and he turned around and headed for me. He actually jumped off the stage, and he found me in the middle of the court. He looked at my camera, wondering if I was going to film him, but

I just held the camera by my side, and I shook his hand. I said: "Good luck." He replied: "Thanks, I'll need it," and that's when it happened. He didn't continue his line of reasoning verbally, but I heard his self-doubt so clearly, and that's where the words ended, but the conversation continued. I looked into his eyes, and my soul talked to his soul. I said, "You are an inspirational leader, and you can definitely become President of the United States of America; you just have to believe it."

"Believe" was actually one of Obama's campaign slogans so obviously he had already heard or been coached to understand the power of belief. But he also obviously needed to act on that knowledge. He had to believe in himself being President. Late that afternoon after the votes were counted, he had won the Iowa caucus, and everyone in the world thought the same thing at the same time: wow, this guy really can become President of the United States of America. And then he did.

When you are meeting a star or someone you really respect, your senses are more awake because it is a very important moment in your life. You step into the Zone, and subliminal communication is more obvious. But you are already communicating subliminally with everyone you meet, and even those you only sometimes see across the room. As you become more awake, you will realize those conversations are constantly going on in your life. President Obama may have had no awareness of that specific subliminal conversation, but it was still happening, just as it also happens for you all of the time.

When I met my wife, Sheila, for the first time, there was an obvious, powerful subliminal connection. I was at a restaurant by the ocean in Santa Monica with my friend, Andrew Wilson, standing by the bar, when I saw her at a table having dinner with her friend, and I intuitively was very attracted to her. I immediately thought to myself I really want to meet her. We connected eyes briefly, but she wouldn't hold onto my stare so when I saw her get up from the table after finishing her dinner, I maneuvered to the entrance. As she brushed past me to leave, I tried to introduce myself, but she wouldn't look at me, and she just walked past. I watched from the door as the valet pulled her car up, and she and her friend drove off. Andrew joined me at the door, and he asked what happened. I admitted sheepishly I had completely choked, and I didn't land a connection. I am usually very open and good at meeting people, so I felt I had really missed an opportunity.

Andrew and I decided to leave, and as we were driving off, he asked if I wanted to drive up the coast to Malibu. He mentioned there was a cool restaurant up there with a very fun bar scene on Tuesday nights, and it was Tuesday. I reluctantly complied, and we started driving up the coast to Malibu. During the drive, all I could think about, and talk to him about, was how I really wish I had met that girl. I told him there was something about her I was really attracted to. Now my wife, Sheila, is a beautiful woman, but it wasn't totally a physical attraction for me; there was something else that attracted me on a deeper level.

We pulled into the parking lot of the restaurant in Malibu, and with a little "luck" we got the last parking space right in front. As I was walking toward the restaurant I had a feeling, and I mumbled, "wouldn't it be incredible if that girl showed up here too?" Andrew replied, "that would be impossible."

As I entered the restaurant, I was immediately glad we came. The place was on fire. It felt so alive and electric, packed with a fun crowd of people, all having a great time. I immediately searched the crowd for her, but she was nowhere to be found. I don't drink alcohol, but occasionally when I am at a bar, I'll really let loose and have a Coke or a non-alcoholic beer. The little bit of caffeine or residual alcohol is not good for your nervous system, but occasionally I revert to my decadent ways.

I turned around from the bar, looked to the entrance, and

there she was, entering. Our eyes connected, and I smiled. I walked straight up to her and said, "So you're following me around?" She laughed and said: "No, *you* are following me around!" and as we both were laughing, I looked straight into her eyes, and I literally fell into her soul. The subliminal connection was so strong – our souls totally connected. We both completely felt it, and instantly I knew she was the girl I was going to marry. She knew it too, and we both spent the rest of the night staring into each other's eyes and talking over our future together. We kept on joking about it because it was so incredible, but we both knew it was true. Sheila and I have now been happily married for 20 years. Yes, there have been a few speed bumps as there are in all relationships, but we are definitely perfect for each other, and we easily recognize it. Our relationship is full of laughter and happiness.

Banfeba Meditation: The Seven Steps

Breathe, Accept, Now, Feel, Experience, Being, Awareness. I named the meditation technique, BANFEBA, to plant the seed of the Seven Steps into the collective consciousness of humanity. From a more personal perspective, I wanted to always remember the Seven Steps, so I created an acronym I could constantly repeat that would immediately trigger the Seven Steps. *The one word – BANFEBA, is all the knowledge we need to remember in life to experience enlightenment.*

Practice the Seven Steps Effortlessly

The purpose of BANFEBA Meditation is to transcend thinking in order to experience Being. Practice the steps until they are done naturally without effort. The Seven Steps need to be done automatically, effortlessly, resulting only in the experience of Being Awareness.

Once you actually start experiencing Being Awareness on a regular basis, the experience will continue to increase. The attraction of pure consciousness to more pure consciousness is exponential. BANFEBA Meditation is a simple technique, but it will lead to a profound transcendental awareness of the bigger, more profound part of you – God.

The Order of the Seven Steps

Although the Seven Steps are linked together and designed to follow a progressive order, *it is not imperative the Seven Steps are always done sequentially*. It is best to start off with deep breathing because until you transcend your thinking the remaining steps will be harder to achieve. Conscious breathing can be done at any time, anywhere, so it is the easiest step to start with. However, once you become familiar with the Seven Steps in the sequential order, if you drop into step two or three without breathing that is fine, or if you feel Being without the first three steps that is fine too. *The goal of BANFEBA Meditation is to Experience Being Awareness.*

There will always be some thinking, intermittently, drifting in and out. The difference is that the thinking doesn't take over who you are, and control you. You will be able to effortlessly escape the thinking, and go to a place where you are just experiencing Being Awareness. Throughout the BANFEBA Meditation process, even over time, you might have the thought – oh, I have to breathe. Or, I have to accept the Now. Or, I want to feel Being. Or, I need to try to be aware of Being. You are skipping steps. That is fine. Those thoughts are fine.

Never fight the thoughts that you are skipping steps – that will only create more thinking. Accept the thoughts. It is a process that takes time to learn. Just breathe, accept whatever comes, feel, and experience it. *You have to continually practice the Seven Steps of the BANFEBA Meditation technique to become enlightened, but you are building habits that will pay off later in an extremely beneficial way, and as you become more and more awake, life becomes better and better at every stage.*

THE SEVEN STEPS

The Seven Steps form a natural progression, and it is important to memorize the order – BANFEBA. However, once you reach a level of awareness that has transcended thinking, and you are constantly Experiencing Being Awareness, you don't need to consciously follow the order of the steps; it will be effortless.

The Seven Steps Will Connect You to Everything in Life

You might be walking down the street, look up, and notice the sky is a beautiful blue. You become aware of it, and immediately feel the bliss of Being. Okay, you skipped a few steps, but it doesn't matter, just keep experiencing the bliss of Being Awareness as long as you can. You don't need to attach a word to it or a belief system. You are already there.

However, if you are standing in a long line at an airport, the bank, a ticket office, or a coffee shop, don't allow yourself to become impatient, or frustrated. Just start the Seven Steps, and work through them methodically, until you are Experiencing Being Awareness, and your experience will be transformed. Soon, you will notice something good is happening, or someone is entertaining, funny, beautiful, or very friendly in front of you in line. You will start to notice this is an exciting moment, alive with possibilities. Enjoy it. Waiting in this line isn't a waste of time. It is like a fun movie, and you are creating it, every second, every minute of every day of your life because you are connected to the Universe. You are connected to the Source of life.

The Power of the Seven Steps

Once you master the Seven Steps, and you are able to return to the Experience of Being Awareness at will, you will become invincible. Someone can be rude to you, treat you with disrespect, or insult you, and it doesn't stick, it just goes right through you, out into the Universe. They are attacking your ego, but you are not identifying with your ego. You are now identifying with and experiencing, Being. Being effortlessly forgives them, and the result is you are invincible to their negative behavior.

Sometimes the negative cycle of thoughts will stick for a few minutes if your encounter is with a family member or a close friend because those situations bring up old, life-long negative patterns of behavior. However, even those strong, challenging feelings will dissipate fairly quickly using the Seven Steps, and you will soon witness yourself from the perspective of Being Awareness, caught in an old game of ego vs. ego.

Most of the time, people will treat you with respect and love because you are always, naturally, treating everyone else with respect and love. You will effortlessly be linking up with good people because you are projecting good energy.

Times might, occasionally, be hard financially, or you might experience a brief period of sickness, but through your connection to Being, using the Seven Steps, financial stability, and good health will return. Being is invincible. Being is infinitely powerful, and through your connection with Being you also have the ability to be infinitely powerful.

The Seven Steps: #1 Breathe

You're headed to an important screening, or a business meeting, or an event, or a party where you will be surrounded by a lot of new people that may dramatically change your life in some way. You have been daydreaming about this event for weeks. The outcome could be extremely positive: an award, a higher position in life, more money, a new job, a new partner, a wife, or a husband. This is a big opportunity for you. You are nervous. You can feel the anxiety building.

This morning your car wouldn't start. It is now in the shop. You had to take the bus. There is more traffic than usual. People seem to be cutting off the bus driver. They are erratic in their driving patterns. The bus driver doesn't seem to be focused either. Your anxiety builds. You are going to be late for your important meeting. If you are late, you will give a bad first impression. This is important. Your mind is racing.

Stop, take a deep breath, and take another breath. Continue to *breathe* deeply. Your thoughts will subside. Every time you feel thoughts trying to jump back in – and they naturally will – take a deep breath, become aware of your surroundings, and recognize you don't really need to do anything right now. *Breathe and Accept the Now; Feel and Experience Being Awareness.*

The Seven Steps: #2 Accept

Accept the traffic, accept the people driving erratically in the path of the bus, accept your feeling of anxiety, and accept the thoughts that drift in and out. Don't fight anything, ever. Just breathe, and *accept* the world you have created. Transcend your desire to succeed in this meeting, event, etc. *Breathe and Accept the Now; Feel and Experience Being Awareness.*

The Seven Steps: #3 Now

As soon as you place your awareness on your breathing, on what is happening around you, you will become aware of what is taking place right *now*. Your desire pulls you out of the Now. Transcend your desire to succeed in this meeting, event, etc. You will become present. Your thinking mind will automatically try to jump back in and analyze your situation. It will take over until you are back lost in thoughts. It will build anxiety and stress. Take a deep breath and accept whatever is happening right now. *Breathe and Accept the Now; Feel and Experience Being Awareness.*

The Seven Steps: #4 Feel

Don't think about what is happening now, just *feel* it. Feeling will keep you in the Now. Feeling will keep you present. Don't think about your anxiety, feel it. Don't think about the sweat rolling down your lower back, feel it. Take a deep breath, accept whatever is transpiring now, and feel it. Feel what is going on inside your body. Feel the energy inside your body. It fluctuates, it moves, it changes. You start thinking, "this is crazy. I'm late!" Take a deep breath, accept whatever is happening now, and feel it. Feeling will allow you to transcend the thinking. Feeling Being will connect you with Being.

You cannot force the feeling of Being. You have to accept the feeling of Being. The more you force the feeling, the more it will evade you. Accept Being, and it will reveal that it has always been there at your Source. *Breathe and Accept the Now; Feel and Experience Being Awareness.*

The Seven Steps: #5 Experience

Very subtly become aware you are the feeling of Being. It is your Source.

Experience Being. *Breathe and Accept the Now; Feel and Experience Being Awareness.*

The Seven Steps: #6 Being

You now feel you are connected to *Being,* the Source of all creation. Feel the loving sensation fill your body. This is now your reality. The tangible experience of this new reality will confirm to you that you are on the right path. *Breathe and Accept the Now; Feel and Experience Being Awareness.*

The Seven Steps: #7 Awareness

Feel and experience Being. Be *aware of* that experience, and now peace, love, happiness, and bliss becomes yours to experience.

THE SEVEN STEPS

Being feels like glowing, pure energy emanating from deep, profound silence. The *Awareness* of that feeling of Being will allow love, happiness, and bliss to now become your experience. Welcome to the experience of enlightenment.

You're still on the bus, on your way to your event. You see trees lined up on the side of the road. You see a mother walking on the sidewalk with her child. Don't think about the trees, and the mother, or the child, just be aware of them, and the experience. Feel Being. Be aware of the experience. It's great. Suddenly, the traffic flows smoothly, the lights turn green in front of the bus, you feel peace and contentment. The sea of cars parts in front of you and the bus pulls over at a stop right in front of your destination.

You glance at your watch. You're right on time. You hop out of the bus, stepping over a puddle, to your event, where someone special notices you arriving, and smiles. You share a story of broken cars and bus rides. You laugh and spend the rest of the event together bonded like great friends, partners, spouses, or lovers. This was the person you were looking for in life. Welcome to enlightenment. *Breathe and Accept the Now; Feel and Experience Being Awareness.*

The Seven Steps: Banfeba Meditation

The Seven Steps of BANFEBA Meditation is a great path to enlightenment, but BANFEBA Meditation is a technique you must practice continuously to master. Sandy Koufax could tell you how to throw a curveball, but unless you practice it continuously, you will never perfect it.

Once you try BANFEBA Meditation and actually experience what is explained in this book, you will know it works. Then it is only a matter of practice. How much do you want to throw a curveball? You don't like baseball? How about tennis? Golf? Surfing? Skiing? How about photography? Guitar? Cooking?

How about life? We all want to live a happy, successful life, full of love, perfect health, beauty, and prosperity. Don't we? BANFEBA Meditation is your ticket. BANFEBA Meditation will bring all of this to you and more. More? How can you want more than that? Your lower self can't even comprehend more, but your Higher Self is infinite. Once you have experienced the slightest taste of infinity, you will know.

Go for a walk on the beach, and see the waves crashing. It is beautiful, and that beauty can change your mood to a happier one, but through BANFEBA Meditation, as you transcend thinking, you not only witness the waves magnificence, you become aware of your oneness with the waves. You are connected to everything you can see surrounding you, and beyond. You are part of the waves, beach, coastline, planet Earth, and the Universe.

The Seven Steps are One Step

The final lesson of learning BANFEBA Meditation is to understand *the Seven Steps are all interconnected and ultimately one step*. When the Seven Steps are each learned so well that they become effortless – they will become one step. When you start experiencing BANFEBA as one step, you will be very close to enlightenment. When the Seven Steps of BANFEBA become one effortless, natural step, on a regular basis, you will be enlightened. You will live your life identified with Being Awareness. You will live your life totally aware that you are an expression of God, and the experience will be absolutely amazing.

The Seven Steps; Time for Meditation

It is optimum if you allow time during each day for ten to twenty minutes where you sit quietly and practice the Seven Steps. You will feel so much better. It will really help you experience Being Awareness. It will also help you practice the Seven Steps as you return to activity.

There will be times in your life, throughout your spiritual journey, that you become overwhelmed by the collective stress you encounter during your daily life. You will feel totally stressed out and irritable. Even if you completely understand every word ever written in all the great spiritual books combined, you may still want to scream. You may even know exactly why you are angry or stressed out, but even that doesn't help. Especially, at these times, you need to sit down in as quiet a place as you can find, and only focus on your Seven Steps. Meditate using the Seven Steps until you can Feel, and Experience Being Awareness. Continue this until the stress has dissipated, then go back out into the world. It may take five minutes; it may take twenty minutes. It might take an hour. You will Experience Being Awareness after you have transcended the thinking mind, and then your natural happiness will return. *Breathe and Accept the Now; Feel and Experience Being Awareness.*

Chapter Nine

Seven Results

PERFECT HEALTH
BEAUTY
PROSPERITY
FULFILLMENT
PEACE
LOVE
BLISS

Seven Steps; Seven Results

BANFEBA Meditation will allow your awakened experience of Being to dramatically support the creation of a healthy, beautiful, prosperous, fulfilling, peaceful, loving, and blissful life for yourself.

    The desire to *create* is a natural part of life. We all have a natural desire to create special experiences in our lives. We are all natural creators. We are part of the expansion of the relative world we live in. Frustration comes when we are not able to succeed in creating what we desire. The reason we are not always able to succeed in creating the life we desire is because we are not awake to the Source of all creation – Being. It is like trying to drive to the store miles away to buy ice cream without getting into the car. We can talk all we want about ice cream, but it's impossible to enjoy unless we hop in the car, and go get it.

The paradox of creating is that in order to create our desires we need to first transcend our desires. You have to transcend your cycle of thoughts. Don't think about your desires. Breathe. Accept everything the way it is. Accept the Now. Feel, and Experience Being Awareness. Your desires will effortlessly begin to be created with a lot less effort on your part. The more you are awake to Being, the faster your desires will be created.

The Seven Steps will help tremendously in allowing your desires to be created. The seven desires mentioned here will begin to be created once you start becoming awake to your connection to the Source, but *any desire* you have will be created if it is in accordance with Being. *Anything that helps you become happier and healthier is in accord with Being.*

Quantum Theory

It is a verifiable truth in physics whatever we focus our awareness on changes in relation to our personal awareness.

Mechanical engineer and physicist, Nikola Tesla, apparently once said, "If you want to find the secrets of the Universe, think in terms of energy, frequency, and vibration." Each of us is conductors of energy. We harness energy, and we send it out into the Universe where it links up with similar energy that is attracted back to us. Our feelings are specifically indicative of the energy we are emitting. Positive feelings are signs of positive energy being released into our world.

The relative world we live in is a maze of streams of energy that flow in different directions with different forces. By constantly using the Seven Steps to experience Being you will always be in touch with an infinite source of positive energy, and that positive energy you project into the Universe will attract more positive energy to you.

Quantum Mechanics and Consciousness

There are theories in quantum mechanics to explain how your actual feelings are created in physical form. If you are interested in researching further, I recommend you study John Hagelin's work on Unified Field Theory. John Hagelin was a researcher at the Stanford Linear Accelerator Center (SLAC) and the European Organization for Nuclear Research (CERN) in the early 1980s. Noble prize winning physicist, Brian Josephson, and several other pioneering scientists have also worked on similar theories. In the science community, these theories are controversial because they are trying to explain a unified field of energy, and its relation to consciousness which is beyond matter and, therefore, by definition, impossible to test in the relative world we live in.

I believe, once again, experience is the only true teacher. The Unified Field as it relates to consciousness is a scientific theory that tries to explain Being, but you won't totally believe it exists until you experience it. You won't completely believe it has the power to create until you personally experience actually creating something physical. Stay awake to the process already happening in your life. Look around you, and let your experience teach you.

You Create Your Reality

Everything in your life: your family, your friends, your house, your car, your clothes, and your bank account all are directly created by your specific thoughts, emotions, feelings, and desires. Being is the Source of it all. It becomes your unique creation because it goes through the filter of feelings you specifically experience. Your unique feelings are an exact frequency of energy.

You briefly dreamed about getting a new watch you saw in a store, but finances are tight, and you need to spend your money on the basics like paying your bills. Your birthday comes around, and it is a big one where there is a zero in your age, so your whole family travels to celebrate with you. You sit down at your birthday dinner in a special restaurant in a special location, and everyone starts handing you gifts. You open the box from your younger brother, and there is the exact watch you had wished for. You are very excited and thank him profusely for his generous gift.

You think back, searching for any clues on how he was tipped off you wanted that particular Swiss Army watch. Even more specifically, how he knew you wanted the Infantry model, but there are no clues because you never told anyone about your desire. You only told the Source.

You may say, oh nice story, but does this really happen? Yes. That literally happened to me. I am now wearing that exact watch my generous younger brother, Hunt, whom I love very much, gave to me on my 50th birthday. It was during a glorious family dinner including my sister, Cam, whom I also love very much, in Big Sur, California overlooking the Pacific ocean at sunset.

It is not just that particular Swiss Army watch I have created. It is literally everything I own – from my Epiphone Casino electric guitar to my house in Santa Monica. It is all so completely specific to the exact desires I've had. It just shows up in my life with very little effort. The material objects, the special events, the special experiences, the special people, everything, just appears effortlessly.

How do you get to the point where you are able to create your desires? *Breathe, Accept the Now, Feel, and Experience*

Being Awareness. When you use the Seven Steps to live in the present moment, you are linking up with Being, which is the Source of all creation in the Universe. The exact scientific explanation of how material objects are created, and situations occur spontaneously in your life may be beyond the human mind to completely fathom because the Source is infinite, but stay awake, and watch it happen in your own life. Jesus said, "If you believe, you will receive whatever you ask for in prayer."[11]

The Stars in Space

The stars may help guide us in life. If you study Vedic Astrology, Jyotish, carefully, I believe you are able to understand the general course you have planned for yourself in this lifetime. Your life will follow a certain pattern guided by the stars. It is a plan your Higher Self, your soul, planned before you came back to Earth in your present life to finish your quest for enlightenment. However, it is important to also understand, you have free will, you can amend that plan, and create any new future you want at any time.

The Stars on Earth

Movie stars, music stars, sports stars, and political stars on Earth are ordinary people just like us. They don't guide us unless we let them. However, because we focus our attention on their lives, they gain more energy from us, and they are able to use that increased energy to create faster. We are able to live vicariously through their glorious, and sometimes perilous journeys in life, and if we are awake we will gain knowledge that can benefit us on our own journeys. We learn to skip mistakes they have made, and conversely, we learn to follow their paths to success.

Each of us creates our own lives, down to every last detail, and the more you are in touch with Being, the faster your desired reality will manifest. We literally create all of our meetings in life, but we may not recognize their significance. Because stars are famous, they are easier to track.

Many years ago, I met Leonardo DiCaprio at a bar in New York City right after he stared in *The Basketball Diaries*. We talked for a while, and I spoke to him extensively about the benefits of meditation. I then told him I totally believed he was going to win an Academy Award some day. It took a while, but he finally did win an Academy Award for his outstanding performance in *The Revenant*. Apparently, he also now meditates.

I also briefly met the director of *The Revenant*, Alejandro Inarritu, at the Director's Guild of America, after a screening of his previous movie, *Birdman*. I shook his hand, and I told him *Birdman* was a masterpiece. I told him he was going to win an Academy Award. Later that night, he won the DGA Best director's award, and then he went on to win the Academy Award for Best Director.

I have a long list of other encounters, and chance meetings I have had with other movie and music stars, and I've got a short story behind each meeting, but the storyline is always the same. I was impressed by each of these artists, and that conscious impression manifested later in a serendipitous meeting. If you look at your own life, carefully, you will see the same thing happening to you. It doesn't have to be a star. We do it with all people we meet. The stars are just easier to track because we imagine more significance in the meeting. But every meeting with every person has significance, and ultimately, every meeting is meant to help guide them and us on our spiritual journeys.

Superman

If you totally believed you could fly, you possibly could, but when you stand on the edge of a huge cliff about to jump, even the slightest amount of doubt could kill you.

Really, fly? There is no scientific evidence of that. It is absurd. Maybe, but my experience has taught me differently. I already told the story of how I literally watched a young man, after meditating for several hours, hang in the air for three seconds, thus defying gravity as modern science usually defines it. That was my experience. He wasn't actually flying, but I witnessed the potential.

Did Jesus really heal people with a single touch? Yes, I believe it is possible he did. He must've done something truly miraculous to become one of the greatest spiritual teachers to ever walk the planet Earth. When your energy is completely in tune with the energy of the Universe, absolutely anything is possible. You become one with the Universe. You can walk on water because you are the water.

I know what you are thinking. You're not Jesus. Well, I am not either. The evidence is clear. I can create $20, playing blackjack in Las Vegas, but if I stepped onto the surface of the pool outside the casino, I would get totally soaked. Why? The same principals are in effect so I should be able to do it. Yes, they are, but our level of awareness is not. Your awareness and your belief are intrinsically tied together. As your awareness expands your experience expands, and then your belief expands, to the point your experience has taught you it is obvious you can walk on water, so you do.

The infinite Source doesn't know the difference between a penny and a million dollars. The Source is able to create a penny or a million dollars just as fast and with just as much effort. We, however, have a different perspective and because of that, there is a big difference in how fast we can create a penny or a million dollars.

A few famous gurus have become rich, effortlessly. Many times they were criticized for it because critics had a mistaken notion, "The meek will inherit the earth," meant the poor will inherit the earth. They forgot to account for meek rich people. The first lesson you need to teach yourself if you are struggling for money is rich people are not bad. Money is not bad. Money is just energy which you either attract or you don't based on your particular belief system.

Enthusiastic Belief Expedites Your Ability to Create

Belief, fueled by enthusiasm, is how most successful people become successful, whether they recognize that strategy or not. Usually, there is a long period of working hard and then experiencing smaller victories that build to bigger victories. The small victory gives them the confidence and belief they can achieve more, so they do. But how did that really happen? Is the Universe keeping score? No, the Universe is giving just as big of an opportunity for you to succeed as it does to very rich and successful people. I know sometimes that does not feel true, but I am certain it is.

My older brother, John, whom I love very much, worked very hard his whole life in school. He ended up going to Stanford, MIT, and Harvard Law School, and afterwards, he started working at a top law firm during the eighties, in New York City. He was paid very well. At the same time, I was a young, struggling filmmaker. I had been a photographer since I was a kid, and I had studied filmmaking for a year at Columbia University, but I never earned my MFA or had much experience, and I was already trying desperately to make a living as a filmmaker. I slept on his coach one winter. He generously would loan me money and buy me dinners.

It was easy to see John had created a completely different world from mine. For him, buying expensive clothes and paintings for thousands of dollars was realistic because he saw a paycheck each week; for me, it was a fantasy. I saw little paydays occasionally when I would finally land a job, but it was always fleeting.

Even when I tried to project the same feeling of success, I couldn't do it. John had climbed up a steep but tangible ladder, step by step, to build that belief. The creative world I had entered had a ladder too, but it was invisible to me, and at that time I couldn't see it yet.

The Irony of Enlightened Creation

Everyone, no matter how successful, is affected by the ups and downs of nature in the relative world we live in. Once successful people finally run into trouble, their mindset changes, and consequently, more trouble follows, sometimes resulting in complete failure.

The key to creating on a regular basis, regardless of the ups and downs of nature, is to escape the effects of karma. *Become unattached to the relative world by transcending the thinking that ties you to it. Become one with Being. Being is not relative; it is absolute.* Become one with being; become enlightened. Then your desires will be created, unaffected by the relative world. Ironically, your desires will most likely then change because your ego is not in control anymore. You don't need to satisfy its unrealistic demands in order to be happy. You are happy without anything at all.

Divine Creation

The Seven Steps are the key to enlightenment. Enlightenment is the key to divine creation. The Source has created everything in existence, including you. In order to create, you need to be awake to Being, the Source, that is always there. When you are totally aware of your connection to Being, divine creation is effortless. You don't have to work hard to achieve anything; it just shows up at your doorstep. You randomly meet someone who wants to hire you for the job you have been dreaming about. You step into a restaurant and meet your future wife or husband waiting for a table in line in front of you. Everything in the entire Universe is completely interconnected and lined up so everything you desire, divinely, manifests effortlessly.

Create Your Destiny; Don't Be Too Serious

Maharishi once remarked, "we have a serious responsibility in life not to be too serious." I love that quote. It is more than just a fun expression describing a way to alleviate stress. It is a truth of life. As kids, most of us are not serious, but as we get older, we gain more responsibilities. We encounter more stressful situations, the stress accumulates within our bodies, and we become more and more austere. We sometimes scold our children for goofing off too much. We think we are justified because we want to prepare our children for the harsh realities of life.

Life is no picnic, and there is no free lunch. Right? Well, for many people I am afraid those clichés are true, and I have compassion for their plight. Life is hard. All you have to do is look at the starving people in the world, the people at war, the unemployed, the sick, the homeless, the people that have to walk for miles each day just to get water. There is probably very little fun in their lives, and it sounds insensitive to say it is all just a state of mind. The truth is a lot of those people are struggling physically and emotionally. It is our duty as fellow human beings to empathize with them and help them as much as possible. At this stage in their lives, nothing would feel better than food, a bed with a roof over their heads, good health, peace, and a job. However, once the basic necessities of life are taken care of, we need to go deep within ourselves. We need to go to the cause of the suffering and fix it there.

The cause of our suffering is a lack of awareness of our inherent connection to Being – God. We have forgotten who we are; it is now time to remember. When you become awake to your natural connection with Being, your experience will teach you – life will be easier, you will be happy, blissful, and nothing is too serious for very long. In that state of happiness, you will be able to create your desires much easier. *Your level of happiness is an indication of your level of awareness of Being.* Have you ever noticed those children who are always playfully goofing off, also tend to always be so "lucky" in life?

Human Beings

It is important on your path to enlightenment to always remember you are a *human* being, and you will always be a human being while you inhabit your physical body. Even after you become enlightened and totally awake to higher levels of consciousness, you will still be a *human* being. Your ego will not completely vanish. It will always be there in the background.

Your ego will contribute to your unique perspective on life. Your ego will help to develop your personality, your character, your likes and dislikes, and the path you choose in life – your career, where you live, what you eat, what clothes you wear, what music you listen to, and who you associate with. The human part of you, most people have defined you by, is mostly created by your lower self – your ego, until you become awake, and then that changes, but it is still there as part of who you are while you remain in your body.

Your Higher Self, Being, is always there, regardless if you are enlightened, or awake to it, or not. Hence, we are all *human beings*. Practically speaking, this means even an enlightened person will still have a human body with human characteristics. An enlightened man or woman will still sometimes get angry or frustrated. He or she may occasionally yell ferociously, or act selfishly, or lustful. This may feel totally contradictory to what we have always thought enlightenment is all about. We may think an enlightened man or woman is so in touch with God they are an expression of God on Earth. They are, therefore, God-like. Well, this is true to a degree. However, this type of reasoning can be misleading, and it has been a major obstacle to reaching and recognizing enlightenment for many spiritual seekers. We judge others, and ourselves, thinking they, or we, can't be on the path to enlightenment. They, or we, just yelled loudly, or got frustrated, or flirted, or acted arrogantly, or selfishly.

The key is to understand you will always be *human* while you inhabit this body and to accept it. This comprehension will help you to transcend your human nature so Being influences every aspect of your human characteristics. You will be guided now predominately by your Higher Self, not by your ego.

Sometimes, however, your ego may return briefly due to old habits or emotional triggers that are still embedded in the background. You still may get angry, frustrated, or feel complacent, greedy, or lustful, but you will not be attached to those feelings, and they won't rule you. You will witness your feelings and actions while simultaneously being awake to your Higher Self, Being, where absolute peace, love, happiness, and bliss constantly remain.

Creation of Collective Egos

We will always simultaneously be the point value (our individual awareness, or Higher Self) and the whole value (Being). While living on this relative plane of existence, we need our individual perspective to remain present on Earth, it creates our physical bodies, but we need to completely transcend our egos influence, so our Higher Selves are guiding us. *Our individual awareness, our Higher Self, our Souls, is ultimately who we are with or without our physical bodies, and that should be our ultimate identification.*

Our thoughts and feelings have created this mental image of ourselves, and referentially all other people on the planet. This mental image becomes our reality. We grow up in families and communities with similar thought patterns and feelings, and those thought patterns and feelings create similar experiences. We dress similar, act similar, think within a certain range or frequency of thoughts, and we are attracted and bonded to each other based on those similar frequencies.

It is no accident you meet someone on the train sitting next to you, and after an hour of conversation, you realize you have a lot in common. That is how we meet our friends, lovers, and everyone within our sphere of existence. We are constantly projecting our thoughts and feelings into the Universe. Those vibrations are linking up with similar vibrations, and those people are showing up in our lives.

If we travel to another country, we notice different cultures with people that seem so different from ourselves. They, however, are only different because they have grown up living with different beliefs. When we start to accept their beliefs, we start thinking like them, we become more like them, and we bond with them. When we, as groups of like-minded individuals, focus only on our differences with other groups, our collective egos fight, and sometimes war is the outcome because we have failed to see the unity of all beings.

Create Miracles

It feels just like yesterday – but it was more than seventeen years ago – I had just finished directing my second movie, *The Last Hand* (aka, *After the Game*), and I was rushing the first edited cut over to the Sundance Film Festival office in Santa Monica, California. I was rushing because it was the last day of submissions for the festival, and I had been working around the clock to get a rough cut ready.

I delivered the film, and I felt this enormous feeling of completion. I was driving back in my old Jeep CJ7 with the top down and the sun shining on me. I remember clearly feeling very peaceful and content.

I was pulling to a stop as the light turned yellow, going up a fairly steep hill, when I looked up to see another Jeep, with a hard top, racing fast down the hill to beat the red light. The other Jeep hit another car that came through the intersection, as their light turned green, and the Jeep flew into the air.

Everything went into slow motion as I instantly recognized the Jeep flying through the air was going to land right on top of me. I turned my head away, bracing for the impact. I distinctly remember calling out in my heart for Jesus to help me, and *I felt this incredibly dynamic sensation of an enormous wave of bright light moving through my body.*

I heard the crash, and I looked right behind me to see the other Jeep tumble twice on the pavement and roll to a stop. I jumped out and raced over. The driver, a teenager, hopped out, bounced to his feet, and miraculously was okay. Several people called the police to stop traffic, and a tow truck to carry away the other, totally smashed, Jeep.

A lady from a car behind the accident approached me like she just saw a ghost, and she uttered incredulously, "Oh my God, the Jeep went right through you!" She declared it was impossible, but she had seen it with her own two eyes; there was absolutely no way the Jeep could miss me. She explained it landed on top of me but went right *through me*. I couldn't prove it, but I came to exactly the same conclusion. I know it sounds impossible, but the Jeep wasn't flying high enough to go over me; it hit me directly, and went right through. My experience was, I actually felt it go through me. I believe it is a total miracle I am alive today.

I realize that story, along with many of my stories, is completely impossible to comprehend, but once your awareness begins to expand, you will start to recognize how the Universe really works, and then you too will begin to believe. I am not Superman. I cannot plan for miracles like this to happen on a regular basis, but my experience has taught me miracles do exist; they are real, and they are happening around the world all of the time.

Create Success Through Enjoyment

Enjoying life is essential to enlightenment. You may be thinking I have the order reversed. You're miserable, even suicidal, you finally surrender to God, you finally let go of your ego-controlled mind, you finally slip into enlightenment, and then you start enjoying life. Well, that path has worked for a few people, but there is an easier, more pleasant way to reach enlightenment. The path to enlightenment is enjoyable, and the enjoyment you are feeling is a good indication you are on that path.

Let's start with step one – you're walking to the store to get some food. You're not hungry, but you're out of the basics: water, bread, rice, beans, vegetables, and you want some cookies. You usually drive to the store, but it is a partly sunny Saturday morning, and you want to get a little exercise.

You walk for a while, and now you're tired. You see clouds in the sky building, and you think it is going to rain. You don't have an umbrella, and you are wearing a new sweater you don't want to get wet, but you are already halfway there, and you figure you have gone too far to turn around. You push the walk sign at the intersection, and you wait patiently as the clouds get closer. The signal changes, but some guy on a bike thinks traffic signals don't apply to him – he comes inches from running you over, and then he acts like it is your fault for getting in his way. You want to scream at his obnoxious behavior, but you take a long deep breath instead.

You're still mad, and it starts to sprinkle as you cross the street. You take a few more deep breaths, watch the biker ride off, and you decide to forgive him. You accept him and the rain. You accept the cards that have been dealt to you right now. You accept the Now, accept the feeling and experience of the Now, feel your feet hitting the sidewalk, and you take more deep breaths. You literally feel your energy change from anger to neutral acceptance.

You cross the street and walk under a line of trees blocking the rain. You look up, and you innocently become aware of the trees. You are walking faster. You look down, and you become aware of the comfortable new boots you bought last week. You breathe again, and you become aware that your body is getting in shape. It is now raining hard, and the streets are empty. You are solo, and it feels good. It almost feels like a dance with you, the trees, and the rain, and suddenly you are glad you walked. You are actually enjoying the rain. Now your sweater is totally wet, but you've accepted that too. You feel the rain penetrating your shirt, but it is okay because this has turned into a special moment.

You look up, as you reach the store, and you see there is a rainbow above it. Is someone talking to me, here? Well, the sun was shining when you started your walk, and anytime there is sunshine combined with rain, there will be a rainbow. You just have to open your eyes, look around, and find it. Will there be a pot of gold? When you start enjoying yourself on a regular basis, you will be amazed at what shows up in your life.

Creating Infinite Realities

If you are at all curious, I am sure you have run across various, strange stories, conspiracy theories, and wild theories throughout your life – Illuminati, the Pleiadians, the Bermuda Triangle, Crop Circles, Atlantis, and countless others. Are any of them true? Yes, to people that believe them, they are true.

If you research the stories in depth, more and more information delivers itself at your doorstep that verifies the reality of the theory. Your thoughts link up with similar thoughts and those build until it literally becomes your reality. Are they real to people that don't believe? No, they aren't. They will look at you like you are completely nuts, but as you reach higher states of consciousness, you begin to witness other frequencies of existence. *Any reality you can imagine is already there. It is your choice whether you want to validate and live that reality, or not.*

Cowboys, UFOs, and the Kennedys

When I was a teenager, age 14, during the radical 70's, a year before I found the higher bliss of meditation, I found Cannabis Sativa. I used to smoke Cannabis searching for a way to transcend the boundaries of my boring adolescent reality. I would surreptitiously blow the smoke out of my bedroom window late at night after my parents went to sleep at the other end of our large, cavernous house, while simultaneously, listening to the Grateful Dead band on my Sennheiser headphones. I remember floating off to sleep many nights with Jerry Garcia still playing one of his long, hypnotic guitar solos.

But just in case my son, Weston, who I love more than anything else in this world, and who is now age 16, is reading this, I want to reiterate our earlier conversation and negate any romantic, drug-fantasy notions. I am not a fan of drugs as a tool to reach higher consciousness. Although Cannabis does have medical benefits in specialized situations, the recreation use has several bad side effects, and the long list of fellow artists and spiritual seekers that have died using other, harder drugs as their tool to get high could cover the north face of Annapurna.

Drugs, however, like the more holistic technique of meditation, do have the ability to sometimes tune you into the Source. The thought seeds that are planted there are powerful, and sometimes those seeds have the ability to come to fruition.

To prove my point: cut to the mid-eighties, when I had a chance meeting with Bob Weir and the Grateful Dead band. Was it a coincidence? No, I created it, just like you have created your life story.

Bob Weir introduced me to John Perry Barlow, who wrote a lot of songs for the band. I immediately liked John. After several long, late nights backstage and at the band's hotel, talking to Bob and John about my first movie, *Real Cowboy*, that I wanted Bob to star in, John invited me to visit him at his ranch for a week in Wyoming where I could work with him on the script's dialogue to get the cowboy twang pitch perfect. At the ranch, they had a little shack in the back where they kept guests. I would write all day while John would work on his cattle ranch.

One day John invited me to ride with him out into the prairie on a fast John Deere ATV to a spot where he explained he once found several of his cows lying dead. Their internal organs had been completely sucked out of their bodies with no holes, gaps, or blood stains. He told me there was also a large round burn mark in the field near the dead cows. There was a police investigation, but it ended up being one big mystery. It was a hell of a story, and it really got me thinking. John, like me, had the big storytelling imagination of an artist, but I could tell by looking into his no-bullshit, cowboy eyes, he was telling the absolute truth.

Many years later I read that same story in *George Magazine*, and I talked to George's editor, my friend from Andover, John F Kennedy Jr., about it. Kennedy had spent time on John Barlow's ranch too, which seems like another totally random coincidence, but nothing is random. We all travel in packs. Our lives are energetically and specifically interconnected. John Barlow had shown JFK Jr. that same spot, and he told him that same story.

Cutting to another twenty years later, after the seed had been planted from hearing John Barlow's curious story; I was preparing to go hang gliding, standing on top of Cagle Mountain. One side of Cagle Mountain overlooks the San Fernando Valley of Los Angeles, and the other side – a vast wilderness area covered with mountains.

I had prepared my hang glider for takeoff, but I had to wait with the other hang glider pilots for the wind to switch directions, from the east over the mountains, to the west coming from the sea. The wind usually switched directions in the late afternoon, during the summer, as the Earth cooled at sunset, so we waited patiently. Like an airplane, it is always important to take off into the wind to gain lift, but it is especially important with a hang glider because there is no engine and, therefore, no thrust to gain lift.

We had been waiting for several hours when all of a sudden I looked up, and I noticed a pack of military jets streaking across the sky. They were flying in a V formation at about 40,000 feet. Several of us watched the jets, commenting on how they seemed to be moving so fast.

Then I saw it – a gigantic silver object. It was as big as the whole pack of jets, and it suddenly appeared flying in front of them. It was as if the light caught it, and I could see it, and then it moved in a different direction, and I could see nothing. It only appeared for about 2-3 seconds, but I watched it stop in mid-air and radically change direction at a 90-degree angle to the left. One of the military jets broke away from the pack and chased after it. It felt like the mysterious, enormous silver aircraft was moving digitally on an orthogonal grid using completely new technology. It definitely wasn't flying like a bird, a hang glider, an airplane, or a jet.

Was it Alien? I don't know. All I could think was if the military had technology that advanced, why are they still flying around in jets? Are there Aliens watching over us, interacting with us? One time someone apparently asked Maharishi if there were Aliens, and he reportedly replied: "Oh yes, don't worry about them, just keep meditating."

When I was at Cornell University I had the pleasure of listening to a lecture by the famous American astrophysicist, Carl Sagan, who was asked if there was extraterrestrial life amongst the billions of stars out there, and he replied, "it would be astonishing to me if there wasn't extraterrestrial intelligence."

If you are curious about the existence of Aliens, just start researching the subject on the Internet, and more and more evidence from credible sources will show up. The same is true for any other outlandish idea or conspiracy.

I have intelligent friends that can talk for hours about the legitimacy of Illuminati and the JFK assassination conspiracy, and it goes on and on. Is it true? It is not true for me because I pay no attention to those conspiracies, but it is true for them. We each create our own reality. Look at your life closely, and you will see the seeds planted early that later became your reality.

My mother, Lee MacWilliams, who I loved very much, was best friends with Betsey Shepard. The Shepard family spent the summers living in Hyannis Port, Massachusetts, and we visited them once when I was a young boy. I don't remember much about that visit, except taking a boat ride across the bay, past a private dock and seeing a bunch of swell-looking kids hopping into a brand new Boston Whaler motorboat. It was the first time I had seen that very cool looking motorboat, and I wanted a ride in one too. I was immediately jealous of these kids; the impression was very strong, and a seed was planted.

Ten years later my dad had become successful in business, and he bought our family a Boston Whaler, and I ended up going to Andover where I met one of those kids on the dock: John F Kennedy Jr. I remember very clearly going to a party the fall of my senior year and seeing this new handsome sophomore surrounded by girls, including my ex-girlfriend, and I remember thinking who is this guy? Then I noticed the monogram sewn into his shirt, JFK, and I thought, great, how do you compete with him? I couldn't, so I accepted him, I became friends with him, and he turned out to be a really nice guy.

Springtime of my senior year, I was walking on campus past the Andover Inn on my way back to my dorm, and John F Kennedy, Jr. was outside the Inn talking to his mother. He introduced me to her, and she invited me to have tea with them. I agreed, and the three of us had tea together at the Andover Inn. She was asking me about my family and my background, and as usual, I peppered the descriptions with a couple of good stories and a few jokes. She laughed, and then she turned to John and said: "Do you know who your friend, Bruce, reminds me of?" John started to brush it off, but then he finally said, "Who?" And that is when Jacqueline Kennedy said: "He reminds me of your father." I almost fell out of my chair, and another seed was planted, deeply.

Cut to two years later, when I transferred out of the Architecture school at Cornell into the liberal arts college where I was majoring in Political Science, and my dad asked me that summer what I wanted to be when I grew up. I looked him straight in the eye, and I said: "I want to be the President of the United States." At first, he said, "You don't want that, politicians are all a bunch of crooks," but I replied, "That's why they need me because I won't be a crook, and I want to help our country."

Secretly, my dad always wanted to be President himself. He thought he had already missed his chance because you have to start wanting it very early in life to allow the time to let it come to fruition, and he was already in his late forties, so he started strategizing how he would launch me instead. He called up his good friend, that was a good friend of George H W Bush at Yale, and he got me working for the Bush election campaign that summer in Nashua, New Hampshire. It was the spring of

1980. I was going to join the grassroots campaign right after my last exam at Cornell, but something else happened instead. The night after my last exam, I flipped a car into a telephone pole, and I almost died.

Now, when I look back, it is very clear what happened. My Higher Self was redirecting me. My ego wanted me to be a Formula One race car driver or President of the United States, to attract the girls like James Hunt and JFK, but my Higher Self, wanted me to become enlightened, so it destroyed my ego to redirect me. I was a pompous preppie with my Andover and Cornell pedigree, and my ego needed to be crushed like a bug, humbled, to see the light – and thank God it was.

I didn't really want to be President. My dad did, and I was trying to please him. I loved him very much, and he was a big influence on me growing up, but I'm not a politician. I'm not even the member of a political party. I am not a Republican or a Democrat. I'm an Independent. *I'm an artist. I'm a filmmaker. I'm a storyteller. I am a spiritual seeker.* But that is why I have met several Presidents and presidential contenders because those seeds were planted, deeply, early in life.

Look at your own life closely, and you will see the seeds that were planted, and how they grew into the life you are now living. We are each the creators of our own worlds. The key is to pick a good life to live, one in accord with your soul's desire. The way to do that is to link up with Being.

Being will guide you to lead a fulfilling life, not one that is directed by your ego. Being may lead you to become President, and if that is the case, then it will be right for you. But Being may also lead you to work at McDonald's. If that is the case, then that will be right for you. You may initially feel like you are not living the life you were meant to live, but as you become more aware of Being, you will experience such incredible happiness it will fulfill you in ways being president of anything never could.

The Seven Results: Perfect Health

Sickness is a condition brought on by being out of balance. When our ego-controlled, thinking minds take over, and an incessant cycle of thoughts pulls us away from Being, we easily spiral into negative thinking patterns that appear in our bodies as stress, sickness, and disease. *The best solution to healing our bodies is to restore our natural connection to Being.* Being always creates our bodies in perfect health. Being knows no other way to create. Being exclusively embodies absolute perfection. If we can remain awake, in a state of awareness of Being, we will naturally live long, healthy, happy lives.

When you become sick, and then you look back at your lifestyle in the previous week you can usually see the culprit. You were staying up late, stressed at work, drinking too much coffee or alcohol, eating unhealthy food, or you got into a bitter dispute with someone. All of these circumstances pull us away from Being because they are not in tune with our natural core. We must avoid these situations to stay healthy.

If you want to maintain good health – eat healthy, organic, non-processed foods. Drink lots of fresh water. Exercise every day. Get plenty of sleep. Work in an emotionally healthy environment. Surround yourself with family and friends that love you, and maintain a positive outlook in life. However, ultimately, always remember the most important prescription for maintaining *perfect health* is to stay in proper balance, by staying aware of Being.

Sounds pretty simple. But then comes the Saturday night, holiday party, and you decide you have earned the right after a long, hard week of work to cut loose, so you have those extra two or three glasses of wine or beer, and a big slice of chocolate cake and you stay up until after midnight dancing and singing at a very loud nightclub.

You wake up Sunday morning feeling tired, but you promised a friend you would play tennis, or go surfing, etc., so you stop first at a Starbucks, grab a large cup of coffee, and a donut, loaded with sugar. You lose your tennis match and become irritated at some of your opponent's calls. Some guy cuts you off on the best wave of the day, and you were sharing evil stares for the rest of your surfing session. There is a traffic accident on the road on the way home, keeping you in frustrating traffic for an hour.

You stop off for a slice of pizza and a beer to avoid the traffic, and when you finally get home, you crash in front of the TV, watching a terrible movie or a big game that your team loses. You awake the next morning feeling tired with a slight sore throat, but you have a big presentation at your architecture firm, so you drink a large cup of coffee, and you rush to work. Your boss and the client are not impressed by your presentation, and they point out several big problems.

By lunch, you are feeling sick. You call in sick the next day, and your boss says – take the rest of the week off, there isn't much work at the office, and he is afraid to tell you he might have to lay you off.

The girl, you were starting to date, reads the writing on the wall, and she decides to jump from the sinking ship. She is twenty-nine. She has a serious career, and she is looking for a "serious" boyfriend. You're feeling rather petulant, and you feel sorry for yourself, so instead of adopting a healthy lifestyle, you slip further into sickness. What started out as a common cold becomes the flu, and it is quickly headed to pneumonia.

You are only 32 years old, and you will survive, but if you are 65, you could be in trouble. As you look at the world surrounding you, you start to focus on all the negative aspects of life. It's been cloudy and raining all week. There is too much traffic. People are rude and selfish. New buildings are being built without regard to the traffic or the environment. Global warming has set off a series of environmental disasters, while political leaders are selling out to big energy companies, and they are not living up to their promises. Education in schools is terrible, and the youth culture is obsessed with violent video games, music, and movies. The Internet is plagued with greedy advertising and rampant, uncontrolled pornography. Sexual harassment charges fill the news. Wars and revolution after revolution are popping up around the world. The Middle East is one non-stop war. Terrorism is everywhere. People are blowing themselves up to make a point. Our culture seems doomed. Cancer and obesity are out of control in America. When did we become so sick and obese?

We started blowing ourselves up, became greedy, became addicted to money and sex, started eating too much, became sick and obese when we lost our awareness of Being. We started thinking negatively too much, and the collective consciousness of humanity has led itself in a negative direction toward destruction. Society is sick. Society is not experiencing perfect health. But we must accept it all, and understand it is all part of the natural cycle. We destroy ourselves to redirect and recreate ourselves. It is nature's way of putting us back on the right path, but we have to be awake to it, or it does little to break the cycle, and it will continue to repeat itself.

Breathe deeply, transcend thinking, accept your sickness, and accept the feeling of your sick body right now. Continue to breathe, accept, and feel your inner body until you begin to feel Being. Experience the good feeling of Being, and continue as long as you can.

Look out the window, it looks like the rain has finally stopped, everything is clean from a week of rain, and now it glistens in the sunlight. The colors of the trees are saturated. You don't have to work today because you don't have a job, so you take a walk on the beach. The crashing waves are soothing. You feel remarkably healthier. You lost weight in your sickness, but you needed to lose a few pounds anyway so this could be a good thing. You stop on the way home, and you have a veggie juice made for you. It gives you a lot of energy, and you are starting to feel like a new man. The radio in the car plays your favorite song.

You get home, check your email, and you see a friend is building a new house, and he wants to know if you are free to design it. This is your chance to break out on your own and start your own company! Things are looking good. Your phone buzzes; it's the girl that just broke up with you, now texting you. She misses you, and she asks for another chance. Go ahead, laugh, yes, the Universe is playing with you. Appreciate it, stay healthy, stay aware of Being. You're on the path to enlightenment.

The Seven Results: Beauty

Perfect health is beautiful. When you are the right weight, in perfect proportion for your body type, and your skin and hair radiate a healthy glow – you are beautiful. When the light in your eyes sparkles, your laughter is full, innocent, and natural – you are beautiful. When anything in the world is healthy, and in balance, beauty is its natural state. The tall trees blowing in the wind in Oregon, the rivers rushing after a spring rain in Maryland, the white clouds floating past the azure-blue sky on a winter day in Montana, the montage of colorful trees in the fall in New Hampshire, the blue waves crashing on the white sandy beach on a summer day in California. America is a beautiful place. The world is a beautiful place. Nature, when it is left alone, is remarkably beautiful. We as a part of nature are naturally beautiful when we don't pollute ourselves with toxins, poisons, and negative thoughts.

When we are aware of Being we are at one with nature, and we will become aware of our bodies in a very healthy way. By choice, we will stop polluting it with cigarettes, drugs, alcohol, fat, salt, sugar, and processed foods. Not because we are feeling remorseful or guilty, but because we recognize how much better we feel without them. We will eat healthier and exercise more because we will feel better.

This all translates to being more beautiful. Your skin will clear up. The bags under your eyes will disappear. Your hair will be full. Your breath and body will smell better. You will be stronger and have more energy. People will be attracted to your charisma. They will want to be in your company. They will want to be your friend. They will want to date you, kiss you, hug you, marry you, and have children with you. Physically, you will be more attractive, more compelling, and your positive energy will attract similar positive, healthy, beautiful people.

During the eighties I lived in New York City. I worked as a film director, and I dated several fashion models. Through them, I was able to look through a window into the fashion world. Admittedly, I was blinded by their seductive beauty for a long time, but one thing has eventually become abundantly clear to me as I have aged in life, and I pulled back the fashion world curtain – true beauty is not a mask of provocative clothes and professional makeup; true beauty is a paragon of perfect health.

True beauty comes in all shapes and sizes. Skinny is beautiful, so is curvy. Tall is beautiful, so is short. Uniqueness is beautiful. If we all walk down the runway of life looking the same height, and the same size waistline, how boring would that be? Perfect health is beautiful in whatever form it comes in. The connection to Being transcends physical beauty. True beauty is absolutely dazzling. *The alluring, dynamic charisma certain people have is their connection to Being.*

For those of you still too cynical to accept my inner beauty paradigm, I have something more obvious for you to get excited about. Most people will agree we were physically more beautiful at age 19 then we will be at age 70. I still believe you can be stunning at age 70, but for those that disagree, I have something that will help you get on board. You will age much slower if you start using a meditation technique. There have been numerous scientific tests done on meditation techniques (specifically, TM) that prove you actually slow down the aging process by meditating.

It works in two ways. The first way is all valid meditation techniques, actually, slow down your heart rate, and give you a deep rest that allows you to physically recuperate. Stress is what ages us, makes us sick, and eventually kills us. Meditation techniques release stress. The second way, which is undoubtedly more esoteric, is that by meditating you will be living more in the Now, and therefore, not subject to the illusion of time. I know this to be true, but I ask you to use your own experience to verify it to yourself. Go meet a group of long-term meditators, and try to guess their ages. You will quickly realize long-term meditators all look much younger than their actual ages. Statistically, long-term meditators live a lot longer than non-meditators by an average of ten years. There have been numerous scientific tests to prove this, but once again, please use your own experience to verify it. You will look younger, be healthier, and have a sparkle in your eyes; that equals captivating beauty.

The Seven Results: Prosperity

Money buys freedom, and we would be lying if we say we don't want to be free. However, the pursuit of money can easily be emotionally bonding, attaching us to a life of strenuous work, disappointment, frustration, and bitterness. Money can be a drug we always want more of. Money can make us selfish. Money can make us greedy and power hungry. So, how do we keep our need and desire for money in proper balance?

First of all, we need to view money from the right perspective. Money is not bad or good. Money is equivalent to energy. It is how we earn it and spend it that makes it bad or good. Can you be very rich and still good? Yes, look at Bill Gates and Warren Buffet, who along with a philanthropic group of the richest people in the world, are committed to giving away billions of dollars to help save our planet.

Let's repeat this one: money has nothing to do with good or bad. Money is only energy. It is how we earn and spend our money that makes it good or bad. We all have heard of extremely rich drug barons that are incredibly evil. The more money you have, the greater the possibilities you have to accomplish benevolent actions and, conversely, nefarious actions. It is not the money that makes someone evil, it is their decadent thought process controlled by their obsessive egos.

When we build our connection with Being we naturally gravitate toward altruistic activities because it is inherent within Being – Being is everything righteous, and nothing negative. Being is always life-sustaining and nurturing.

Our connection with Being will also allow us to create our desires. If you want to earn enough money to buy yourself a beautiful house for your family to live in, and enough money for your children to go to a great college, and you want to buy pure, healthy food – I believe all of those things will come to you fairly easily, because we all believe they are justified.

If you want to buy a Gulfstream jet to impress your mistress on the way to your third mansion in the Hamptons, it might be harder to effortlessly attract the money because we easily recognize it doesn't feed the Universe. However, after connecting to Being on a regular basis, if your intentions are properly aligned, and if you still want it – you may get it. My guess is, at that point you won't really want it anymore, but it's your call; there are no referees in Heaven keeping score. You are the referee. You make the choice, and whatever energy you send out into the Universe links up with similar energy, and it is attracted right back to you.

Maybe you want a beautiful silver Aston Martin? It's a great car. My dad always wanted one, and it reminds me of him. Is it a sign of conspicuous consumption? Only if you believe it is. The Universe knows no difference between a brand new Aston Martin and a rusty old Fiat. Only we do, so we place limits on ourselves. Do I own an Aston Martin? No, it's pretty far down my list of desires, but maybe someday I will. Pick any car, house, and future you want. It's your call. Just remember, if your ego wants to create something, it is much harder. If Being wants to create something, it is effortless.

The Seven Results: Fulfillment

Fulfillment is an extremely pleasant feeling because it allows you to feel deep peace. However, fulfillment doesn't necessarily have to be a feeling you gain only after achieving success. Be careful not to associate the feeling of success with fulfillment. Feeling successful is the ego feeling gratified, and that feeling will always be temporary. The feeling of true fulfillment is felt when you break free from the constant chain of desires. That continual link of desire after desire created by the ego is so tiring, frustrating, and stressful. Desires will never be continuously, instantly satisfied, and anytime a desire is not satisfied, stress will build up in your nervous system.

True fulfillment is a feeling of complete satisfaction that becomes your reality when you Experience Being Awareness. *True fulfillment is a sense that the very moment you are living right now is a phenomenal moment, and no other moment is going to be better.* You still make plans and have future events you look forward to, but each moment is now so satisfying you won't project your happiness into a fictitious exciting future because you are so happy right now. The irony is when you start feeling so fulfilled and happy in the present moment, all of your past ambitions begin to be realized, and you will become more successful.

The Seven Results: Peace

At the core of Being, is a peace that is so deep and so profound, you feel as if you could cut stairs into it and walk up into Heaven. This totally fulfilling peace is so strong it can calm any mood, feeling, or emotion. Once you experience this deep peace, you always want more. The good news is the peace of Being is infinite and eternal, and you can be constantly aware of it.

Your life situation may take you to different places. You may have some euphoric emotions, and some uncomfortable emotions, but the deep peace of Being will always be available to you, and it will naturally be your predilection to feel the peace of Being, instead of the turbulent feelings and emotions of the relative world.

That ability to always feel deep peace is priceless. There is nothing on Earth more valuable. It is so sensually satisfying you don't really need to do anything else in life to keep yourself happy. You probably will do a lot of things, you will accomplish much, and you will have a very rewarding life, but when merely sitting in a chair, looking out a window feels so great, everything else is a bonus.

Prophecy: By Discovering Individual Peace We Will Transcend Ultimate Destruction

Humanity is now at a time in our evolution where constant fighting has potentially reached its zenith, and the ultimate destruction of our planet, as a result of nuclear war, is a very real possibility. Turn on the news. North Korea, with its new ICBM capabilities, is threatening to totally annihilate the United States of America. As I write this chapter, America, has three aircraft carriers, and a submarine armed with ballistic missiles with nuclear warheads, in the South China Sea, practicing a pre-emptive strike against North Korea. It may all be just posturing or a bluff, but no matter how we justify it or rationalize it, we have to realize we are precariously close to massive destruction on planet Earth. And that is just one potential conflict currently on Earth; there are several other potential conflicts also being played out with nuclear-armed adversaries.

The collective consciousness of the world is at a crossroads, and we are starting to head down the wrong path in many ways. War is only one possible threat. If we don't blow ourselves up, Mother Nature may obliterate us in self-defense. Look at what pervasive pollution is doing to our planet, Earth. Look at the recent weather patterns. The increase of hurricanes, floods, and earthquakes are not random. Everything in nature has a cause and effect. Yes, we need abundant energy to run our advanced civilization, but our particular fuel choices have completely polluted our planet. We could have switched course and developed new technologies years ago, but oil and coal continue to make a lot of people extremely rich. Oil and coal were beneficial in their place and time. America was built on the back of oil and coal, but now we must move on. Current adverse weather patterns are a result of our egos running rampant, and blind greed.

If you want to know how healthy a family is, look at the parents. If you want to look at how healthy a country is look at its leader. This isn't a matter of politics. Look at all the world's leaders across the spectrum of diverse ideologies. The world is completely divided. The world is sick. History should have already taught us when conflicting ideologies reach such a paramount level, destruction is inevitable. But we can't fix these problems from the outside. We can't legislate them. We can't dictate them. We can't negotiate them. The world is sick, but we have to heal from the inside out. *Each of us, individually, has to become healthy, and the only way to become truly healthy is to become awake.* It is 2018 AD. Jesus was teaching us the same lesson 2018 years ago. Many other teachers have pointed us in the same direction throughout the history of mankind. We have been in school for a very long time. Now is the final exam.

The good news is, although the media doesn't spotlight this because it doesn't sell as well as fear, we are also actually simultaneously evolving as a species in a positive direction. Many different people, from different cultures, from different countries on Earth, have become more aware that we are, each of us, connected on the soul level. The exchange of spiritual knowledge through the internet is unprecedented in the history of humanity. We are all, around the world, talking to each other, and as the knowledge of enlightenment continues to expand it will guide us to the actual experience of unity.

Once that level of awareness expands more each day because people like you meditate to broaden your awareness, that level of awareness will reach a tipping point, and when enough people on Earth become awake to the reality of our unity, we will become healthy, and there will be peace. *I believe the omnipresent experience of unity will be the next stage of our evolution, and once that occurs, Earth will return to its natural balance, and there will be total peace on Earth.*

The Seven Results: Love

Love is the experience that emanates into the relative world from the absolute peaceful core of Being. Love is the glue that unites everyone, and everything in the Universe. When you are totally aware of Being, in a state of Unity Consciousness, you love everyone and everything. You drive down the road of life, loving everything in sight.

True love is not possessive or conditional. True love is unconditional. You see the good in others, and you love that. Forgiveness and acceptance are automatic and effortless. It is a beautiful experience to be in complete contact with the love of Being. It is hard to explain the experience without sounding artificial, and there is no way to truly believe it until you experience it, but it is incredibly exhilarating.

The Seven Results: Bliss

For me, personally, *bliss* has always been such a pristine word. It almost sounds too good to be true, but you can actually live in a state of bliss. *Bliss is a state of refined happiness so sublime no other experience tops it.* When you experience bliss, it feels like intense happiness, peace, fulfillment, love, and laughter all combined into one magnificent feeling. The uninterrupted experience of Being expresses itself as bliss in the relative world.

Bliss is the goal. There is no higher experience here on Earth. Bliss has different levels of intensity, but the experience is always absolutely amazing. When someone is experiencing bliss, you can easily read it in his or her eyes. There is so much Universal energy moving through them their eyes look like sparklers.

When someone tells you a funny joke, or you see a funny movie, you may laugh at the situation, but when you feel bliss you just start subtly laughing or smiling, and no one did or said anything funny. The blissful experience of Being feels so wonderful you want to smile from ear to ear and chuckle to yourself.

The experience of bliss is so sublime it is hard to explain in words. I can only say, sincerely from the bottom of my heart, it is worth seeking with every last breath of your life. BANFEBA Meditation *is a technique that allows you to maintain your awareness of Being and establish yourself in a state of bliss.* I have a profound intuitive feeling it will work very well for you. *Breathe and Accept the Now; Feel and Experience Being Awareness.*

EPILOGUE

Jesus, Moses, the Giant Indian, and the Dolphins

My intelligent editor, Julie Civiello, has a talent for catching grammar problems and punctuation mistakes. I look at my script, or manuscript, several times, and I think it is ready to go out the door. I'll hand it to Julie, and she hands it back a few weeks later covered in red ink.

The morning of the day I received Julie's notes on this book, I stopped by Whole Foods to get a banana and strawberry smoothie. As I approached the cashier at the checkout stand, I noticed he was quite unique. He was a young man, handsome, with long blond hair, a beard, and piercing green eyes. I recognized a specific Vedic Mandala tattoo on his forearm. I frequently used to spontaneously doodle that same iconic sign when I was about his age. I later found out it was an ancient sign of God. I immediately felt a connection on the soul level with this young man, and I knew I had some specific knowledge to give to him, but I was unsure exactly what it was.

Later, that afternoon as I was cooking an early dinner of vegetable fried rice for my son, Weston, the doorbell rang. I turned off the stove, and I hustled to the front door. The UPS man, Victor, is a regular visitor to our house, especially during film awards season when us members of the Directors Guild of

EPILOGUE

America receive DVD copies of 10-15 movies, that are trying to earn our votes to get nominated for the DGA Best Director Award, which is a precursor to the Best Director Academy Award. When I opened the door and saw Victor holding a package I knew it wasn't the usual envelope carrying a DVD because awards season hadn't started yet, and it didn't look like the normal boxed package from Amazon Prime either that is constantly showing up at our door for my wife, Sheila. At first, I thought the package was a script, but it felt too heavy. I didn't have my glasses with me so I couldn't read the return address.

After Victor hopped back into his big, brown UPS truck and drove off, I retrieved my glasses. I saw Julie's name on the return address of the package, and I smiled knowing it was her notes on this book. I dropped off the book on my bedside table so that I could review it later, and I went back to the kitchen to finish cooking the sumptuous feast for Weston and myself.

That night, Sheila had fallen asleep on the couch in the living room after watching TV. It was a regular habit of hers. She was comfortable and covered with a blanket, so I let her sleep, and I retreated to the bedroom, alone. As I was about to go to sleep, the encounter with the young blond man that morning came back to me. I felt the meeting was, for some unexplained reason, spiritually significant, and I asked God for guidance on how I could help this young man. I meditated for about twenty minutes, then I fell asleep.

I awoke in the middle of the night. The room was dark, but there was enough moonlight to see. Suddenly, I gasped, as an enormous man, a giant American Indian, walked quickly through the bedroom door – literally, *through* the actual door. I called out in fear for Jesus's help. This was not a dream. This giant Indian was literally there in my room. He was so big he had to bow his head not to hit the ceiling. He stopped only feet away from me, lying in bed. He had long black hair and a weathered face. He was wearing a fedora and a jacket. He was strong and massive, but I calmed down as I realized he meant me no harm. Intuitively, I picked up on the fact he was a spiritual guide, sent by God to help, but I was unsure what he was there to tell me. He looked several times directly at the big leather chair next to the window where I always write, so I knew he wanted me to write something, but I was unclear what I was to write. He then looked over next to me several times as some sort of an indication of what I should write.

He then literally disappeared, vanishing back into the darkness of the night. I stayed awake for a bit longer, absolutely amazed by this incredible encounter. I have not had a spirit visit me like that in more than twenty-five years since the visit from Jesus. I asked God what this giant Indian spirit guide was trying to tell me.

I fell back asleep, and I had a very clear, lucid dream. In the dream, I ran into the young, blond man with the beard, and as I approached him, I saw Jesus and Moses both leave his body and walk off. I tried to tell the young man he was being directly guided by God, but the words wouldn't come.

I woke up the next morning, and I tried to piece together what I was being guided by God to do. The young blond bearded man, who represented many spiritual seekers I meet now more and more frequently, was looking for spiritual guidance. That was obvious to me. The giant Indian spirit guide was telling me to write something that could help the young blond man, but what? I looked to the chair the giant Indian keep gesturing towards. I followed his eye-line to my bedside table, he was also gesturing toward, and there lying on the table was the manuscript for this book. *The Giant Indian Spirit Guide was sent from God to tell me to finish this book.*

I had been procrastinating. I had delayed finishing this book for months. I was looking for a sign it was ready to be released

EPILOGUE

to the world. I got the sign to keep writing and finish the book as a spectacular message – directly from God. But for some unexplained reason, I still wasn't ready. I knew I was close to being finished, but something was still bugging me. Something wasn't right. I couldn't figure it out. Several more months went by, and the book sat there unfinished.

One sunny day I had lunch at my favorite Indian restaurant, Chandni, in Santa Monica, and afterwards, I took a walk in the park on the bluff overlooking the beautiful Pacific Ocean. As I was walking, I clearly heard a word from my spiritual guides, "awareness," and I realized I was totally awake simply to my awareness. I was happy and content simply to be aware without any thoughts. I had no desire to achieve anything. I felt completely fulfilled.

I looked out to the glistening ocean, and there was a pack of dolphins, circling, swimming very close to the shore. That's when I had the epiphany that Awareness was my Seventh Step. Awareness was my final step. Awareness of Being; Awareness of Being, just as it already is, without any desire for anything to change. Awareness of Being leads directly to love, happiness, and bliss.

I could hear the Dolphins. I could feel their pristine energy. I knew they confirmed what I felt, as they played in the ocean, welcoming me to play on a spiritual plane with them. I felt Jesus walking with me on a transcendent plane.

I experienced a complete union with God. *Being* is omnipresent. *Being* is ready. *Breathe and Accept the Now; Feel and Experience Being Awareness.*

NOTES

1 Beveridge, W.I.B., *The Art of Scientific Investigation*, 1957 (Cambridge University professor W.I.B. Beveridge, public library; public domain)

2 Thomas Jefferson, *The Jefferson Bible*, (Dover Publications, New York, 2006), p 23.

3 Thomas Jefferson, *The Jefferson Bible*, (Dover Publications, New York, 2006), p 19.

4 Thomas Jefferson, *The Jefferson Bible*, (Dover Publications, New York, 2006), p. 25.

5 Pogrebin, Robin (2007-01-14). "Art," New York Times.

6 Max Planck, *Where is Science Going?* (Ox Bow Press, 1981)

7 Walter Isaacson, *Einstein: His Life and Universe*, (Simon & Schuster, New York, 2007)

8 Buettner, Dan, "The Secrets of Long Life.", National Geographic, November 2005. P. 9.

9 Ephesians 3:16, (International Version of the Bible)

10 Mark 9:23, (International Version of the Bible)

11 Matthew 21:22 (International Version of the Bible)